The Anthropocene: Politik—Economics—Society—Science

Volume 12

Series editor

Hans Günter Brauch, Mosbach, Germany

More information about this series at http://www.springer.com/series/15232
http://www.afes-press-books.de/html/APESS.htm
http://afes-press-books.de/html/APESS_12.htm

Lydia Wanja Gitau

Trauma-Sensitivity and Peacebuilding

Considering the Case of South Sudanese Refugees in Kakuma Refugee Camp

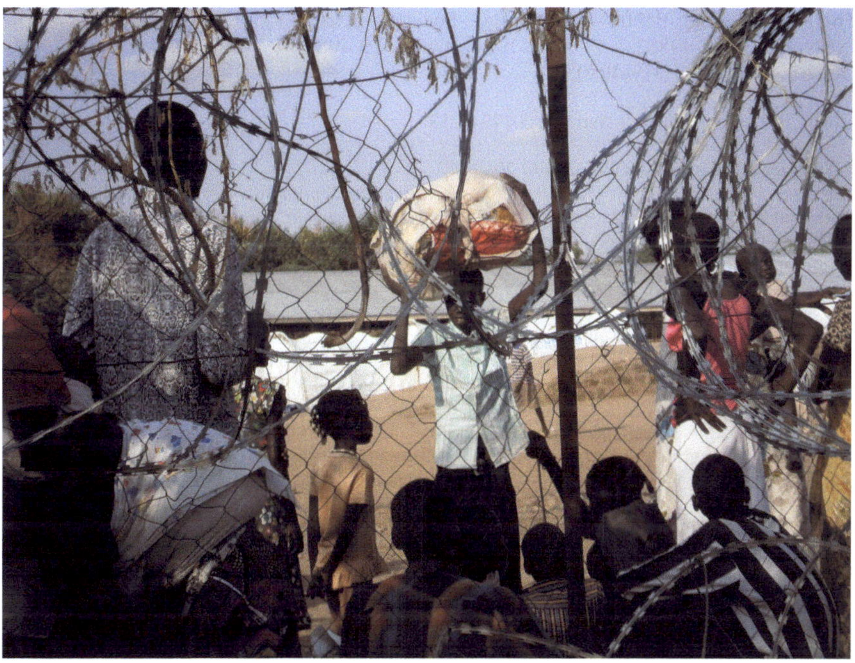

Springer

Lydia Wanja Gitau
Centre for Peace and Conflict Studies
University of Sydney
Sydney, NSW
Australia

This research was funded by the Peace Research Grant Program of the International Peace Research Association Foundation, and the University of Sydney's Postgraduate Research Support Scheme.
More on this book is at: http://afes-press-books.de/html/APESS_12.htm

ISSN 2367-4024 ISSN 2367-4032 (electronic)
The Anthropocene: Politik—Economics—Society—Science
ISBN 978-3-319-49802-7 ISBN 978-3-319-49803-4 (eBook)
DOI 10.1007/978-3-319-49803-4

Library of Congress Control Number: 2017943253

Cover photo: Newly arrived refugees at the Kakuma Refugee camp Reception Centre: *Source* The Author. The photo on page 87 shows a refugee posing with some samples of her embroidery work. *Source* © The Author. Photo used with permission from Teresa Achol.

Copy-editing: PD Dr. Hans Günter Brauch, AFES-PRESS e.V., Mosbach, Germany
Style and English Language Editor: Dr. Ken Macnab, Centre for Peace and Conflict Studies at University of Sydney, Sydney, Australia

Printed on acid-free paper

This Springer imprint is published by Springer Nature
The registered company is Springer International Publishing AG
The registered company address is: Gewerbestrasse 11, 6330 Cham, Switzerland

This book is dedicated to those
Who have watched their homes shattered
And seen their loved ones murdered
Suffered the agony of wars they did not allow
Scampered for safety in places they had not foreseen
And are begrudged a location on this earth.
'Peace is you'.

Acknowledgements

I would like to express my special appreciation and thanks to Dr. Wendy Lambourne and Prof. Paul Rhodes of University of Sydney, and Dr. Lucy Fiske of University of Technology Sydney, for your academic mentorship and support through my research journey, culminating into the writing of this book. My sincere thanks go to my colleagues at the Centre for Peace and Conflict Studies, University of Sydney, and especially to Dr. Ken Macnab for thoroughly going through the entire manuscript and for your invaluable advice, and Emeritus Professor Stuart Rees for your inspirational passion for peace.

My special thanks go to the Kenya Department of Refugee Affairs, the LWF leadership and the team in Kakuma for allowing me to do my research in Kakuma refugee camp, and for the support they offered me. A very special thanks to all the refugees I interviewed in Kakuma, for so generously sharing your stories with me. Your stories have remained with me, and I have been greatly challenged and encouraged by your courage and hope. I am very grateful to you. I would also like to heartily thank the International Peace Research Association (IPRA) Foundation, for granting me the 2014–2015 Dorothy Marcus Senesh Postgraduate Fellowship, which greatly assisted me financially towards my research, and the University of Sydney for the Postgraduate Research Support Scheme grant.

Most specially, I would like to thank my family. Thank you Gitau for being loving and supportive, and offering very insightful thoughts to my work. Thank you to our children Hadassa and Mwenda, for your patient understanding, your interest in my work, and enthusiasm in life. You inspire me. Thank you to my Mom, Elizabeth Wangari, and my mother-in-law Rosemary Wangui, for your prayers, love and concern.

Thank you to all my friends for walking with me through the journey. Special thanks to you Leah, for your daily encouragement, counsel and prayers. And thanks to my church family in Riverstone, Sydney, for your love and support. Indeed, thank you to everyone who helped me in any way through this journey. I am thankful to God for all of you, and I thank him for succour that sustained me through it all.

Sydney, Australia Lydia Wanja Gitau
March 2017

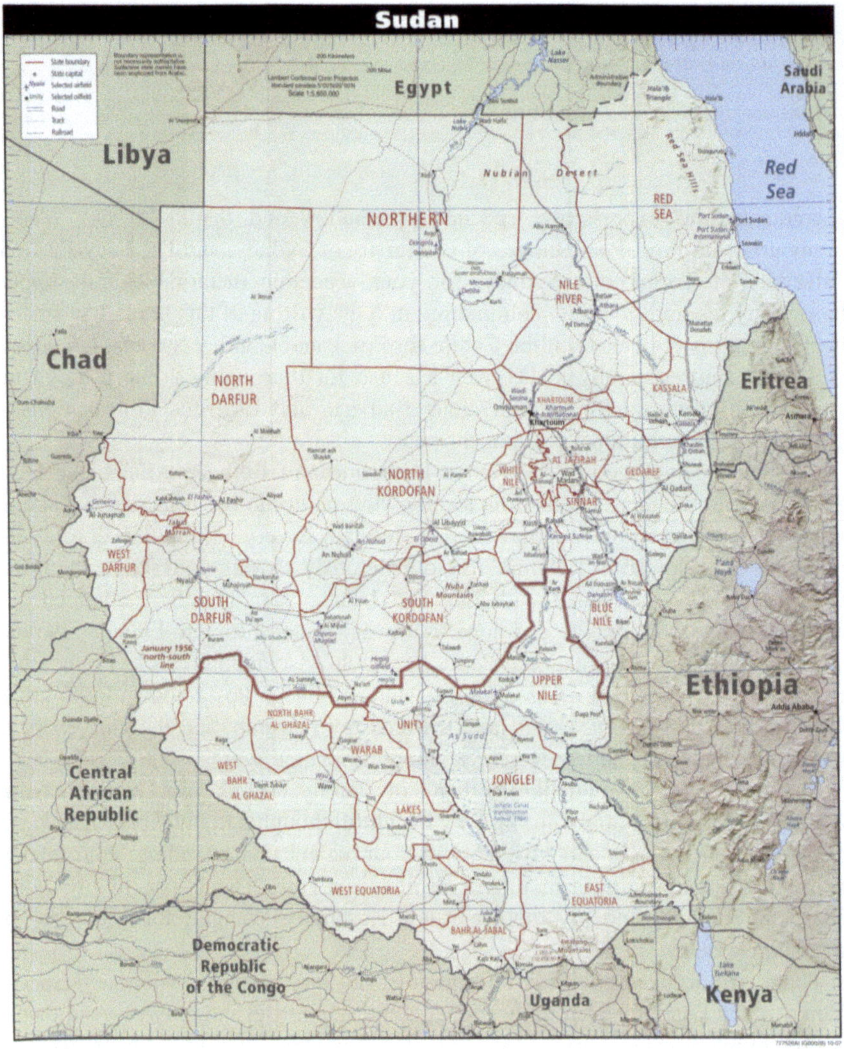

Map 1 Map of Sudan: *Source* Library of Texasa Austin, Perry-Castañeda Library Map Collection; at: http://www.lib.utexas.edu/maps/africa/txu-oclc-219400066-sudan_pol_2007.jpg. Free use of maps that are not copyrighted based on conditions that are at: https://www.lib.utexas.edu/maps/faq.html

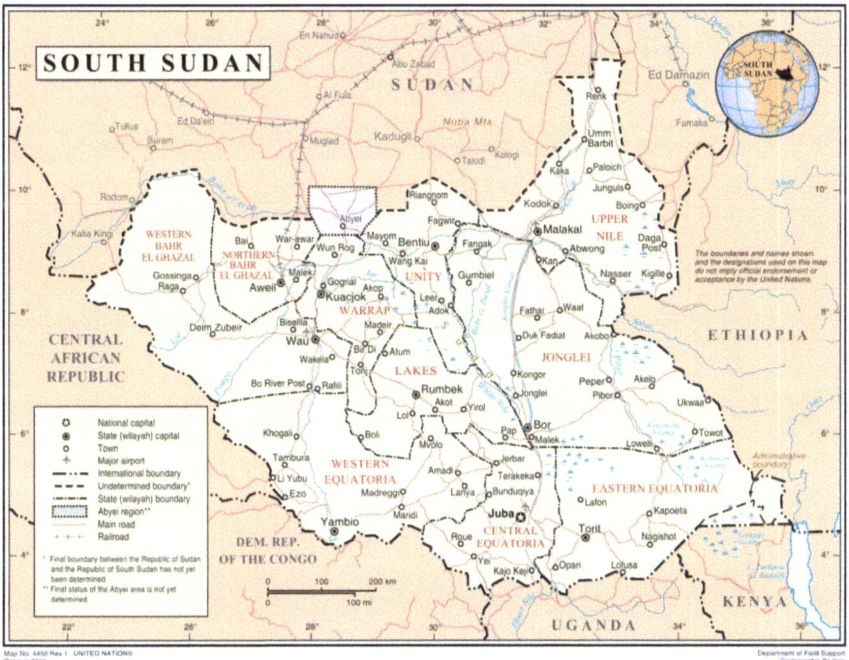

Map 2 Map of South Sudan. *Source* United Nations, Department of Field Support, Carthographic Division, Map No. 4450, Rev. 1 (October 2011). Permission was granted by the UN Carthographic Division

Contents

Abbreviations and Acronyms

AI	Appreciative Inquiry
APA	American Psychiatric Association
APT	Amani People's Theatre
AU	African Union
CARE	Cooperative for Assistance and Relief Everywhere
CEWARN	Conflict Early Warning and Response Mechanism
CPA	Comprehensive Peace Agreement
CPT	Choosing Peace Together
CRM	Community Resilience Model
CRS	Catholic Relief Services
CTR	Catastrophic Trauma Recovery
DNA	Dialogical Narrative Analysis
DO	District Officer
DRA	Department of Refugee Affairs
DRC	Democratic Republic of Congo
DSM	Diagnostic and Statistical Manual
DSM-IV-TR	Diagnostic and Statistical Manual of Mental Disorders, Fourth Edition, Text Revision
EU	European Union
GPI	Global Peace Index
HIV/AIDS	Human Immunodeficiency Virus/Acquired Immune Deficiency Syndrome
IASC	Inter-Agency Standing Committee
ICG	International Crisis Group
ID	Identity Card
IDP	Internally Displaced Persons
IGAD	Intergovernmental Authority on Development
IJR	Institute for Justice and Reconciliation
IOM	International Organization for Immigration
IRC	International Rescue Committee

IRIN	International Regional Information Networks
JRS	Jesuit Refugee Services
LWF	Lutheran World Federation
MHPSS	Mental Health and Psychosocial Support
NCA	Norwegian Church Aid
NCP	National Congress Party
NGOs	Nongovernmental Organizations
PTSD	Posttraumatic Stress Disorder
RSD	Refugee Status Determination
SPLA	Sudan People's Liberation Army
SPLA/M	Sudan People's Liberation Army/Movement
SPLM/A—IO	Sudan People's Liberation Movement/Army—In Opposition
SWAN	Sudan Women's Association in Nairobi
TPO	Transcultural Psychosocial Organization
UK	United Kingdom
UN	United Nations
UNESCO	United Nations Educational, Scientific and Cultural Organisation
UNHCR	United Nations High Commissioner for Refugees
UNICEF	United Nations Children's Fund
UNMIS	United Nations Mission in Sudan
UPR	Unconditional Positive Regard
US	United States
USD	United States Dollar
WFP	World Food Programme
WICP	Welcome and Information Project
WTF	War Trauma Foundation
WUSC	World University Services of Canada

List of Figures

Introduction: Starting the Journey

My interest in researching and seeking to understand the situation and experiences of the South Sudanese began in 1995 when I visited Khartoum and interacted with people of South Sudanese origin then living in Khartoum, Northern Sudan, many of them displaced due to the conflict in South Sudan. The interest was nurtured over the years as I interacted with South Sudanese refugees living in Kenya, and further established during a training session on trauma recovery that I participated in at Dadaab Refugee Camp in Northeastern Kenya in October 2011, which involved some South Sudanese refugees. In order to understand the experiences and situation of South Sudanese refugees better, I chose to conduct research in Kakuma Refugee Camp, due to its concentration of refugees from South Sudan.

This book examines the traumatic experiences of the South Sudanese refugees, the interventions they receive in Kakuma refugee camp, and the link between those interventions and peacebuilding. In exploring the relationship between trauma and peace for the South Sudanese refugees in Kakuma, this book discusses how a focus on the victims, what they have suffered, and how their pain and anguish can be appreciated and alleviated, is of paramount importance to peacebuilding and can augment current strategies towards sustainable peace.

The research on which this book is based was carried out using semi-structured interviews with South Sudanese refugees in Kakuma. The interviews consisted of a framework of themes to be explored and a number of guiding questions, and were open to new ideas arising as a result of what the participants said. The design of interviews was informed by the interpretivist theory of social science which pays attention mainly to the context of events and meanings of phenomena (Denscombe 2003, p. 280). Principally, Denzin's (1989) concept of *interpretive interactionism* informed the interview design. This is a mode of qualitative research that seeks to capture the voices, emotions and actions of those studied, and to understand their individual and anecdotal experiences. In his approach, Denzin is interested in the interrelationship between 'private lives' and 'public responses' to personal troubles, and emphasizes the uniqueness of each individual life.

The guiding questions asked of the participants were open-ended, to create space for the participants to narrate their experiences (Galletta 2013). The questions sought to capture the participants' voices and emotions. They did not follow a given fixed format, but generally covered the following topics:

- The experiences of war that led the refugees to come to the camp
- How the refugees coped with these experiences before coming to the camp
- What interventions they had received in the camp to help them cope with these experiences
- What the refugees thought about these interventions. How they felt the interventions had helped them cope, or not, with dealing with their experiences
- The refugees' definition of peace
- What the refugees perceived to be the relationship between peace and the interventions they were receiving.

The data gathered in these interviews was analyzed using two methods: Firstly, grounded theory with phenomenology as the underlying philosophy, and secondly, narrative inquiry. The first method involved seeking to grasp the experiential world of the participants of the research, and trying to understand how they were making sense of their world (Smith and Osborn 2003). The key focus was the individual, anecdotal experiences of the participants. Secondly, a subset of five interviews was analyzed using the narrative inquiry analytic procedure as applied by Frank (1995, 2010). Narrative inquiry was chosen because of its value in allowing the voices of the participants to permeate through the book and hence have control of the interpretation of phenomena.

Stories with a plot line; a beginning, middle and an end were constructed from the selected interview transcripts, ensuring that they maintained the chronological aspect, a narrative flow and the voice of the participants (Dawson, Rhodes and Touyz 2014). The stories were then analyzed using Frank's (2010) Dialogical Narrative Analysis (DNA), which maintains that no story has a singular voice, and no speaker should ever be 'finalized' (Frank 2010, p. 16). DNA, as Frank (2010) explains, is a way of questioning that studies the relationship between what is told in the story, and what happens as a result of telling that story. Rather than a set method or rules to be followed, this type of analysis employs 'movement of thought' (Frank 2010, p. 73) which happens in the interaction between the researcher and the participants, 'as those participating in research are given scope to upset the presuppositions of the researchers'. Participants are seen as the experts of their own lives, and the researcher as learning from them.

The analysis sought to uphold the three basic principles of DNA, namely *non-finalizability*, *second person address*, and a *commitment* to not speak a single word about the participant that the participant could not have said about himself or herself (Frank 2010, pp. 99–100). This involves a responsibility to not speak the final word about the participant. Each of the stories chosen has no conclusion. Each is a journey, which even at the end of what the participant relates, seems to continue. No word is pronounced to finalize or end it.

This book depicts a twofold journey: a journey towards an understanding of the crucial role of trauma-sensitivity in peacebuilding, and the journey the South

Sudanese refugees in Kakuma have taken fleeing violence in their country and trying to find refuge and solace for all that they have suffered, and eventual peace. It is a long, tedious, seemingly interminable journey, replete with indescribable perils, hurtful betrayals, countless uncertainties, dramatic turns, and incredible hope.

The first part of the journey, portrayed in Chap. 1, lays out the setting. It describes where the survivor of the conflict is coming from, and why. It describes the context of the conflict in South Sudan, and the decades of war that have led to the situation the survivor finds himself/herself in today. It explains the context of the research, Kakuma refugee camp. It also locates a place for you and me, and our participation in the unfolding of this journey.

The second part, Chap. 2, lays out the bridge that needs to be crossed to get to the desired destination, the gap that needs to be filled if the sojourners are to reach their destination.

It discusses the inadequacy of past and current peacebuilding efforts and the shift of focus to the link between peacebuilding and psychosocial interventions. It also reviews a cross-section of studies that have sought to link peacebuilding and psychosocial interventions, and identifies a place for this book in establishing this link.

The third part of the journey, depicted in Chap. 3, sets out the terrain. It lays the definitional background of the experiences of survivors of violent conflict of whom the South Sudanese refugees in Kakuma Refugee Camp are an example. It predicts both what the survivors will encounter in their journey towards peace, and what we will encounter in our journey towards discovery of trauma-sensitivity in peacebuilding. It prepares the survivor, and us, for the perils, betrayals, uncertainties, surprises and hope that lie ahead. The chapter explores the concepts of trauma, peace and peacebuilding, and specifically addresses the controversies surrounding the meaning and experience of trauma, the definitional fogginess of the concept of peace, and the multifaceted process of peacebuilding.

Chapter 4 invites us to consider where the survivors are at present and reflect back on where they have been in the past. This chapter looks at their traumatic experiences back in their country of origin, on their journey in search of refuge, and in the refugee camp where they are now living. The chapter focuses on the experiences as related by the participants, the meaning they give to the experiences, and discusses these experiences and perceptions in the light of literature and scholarship in the field of trauma and mass violence.

Chapter 5 continues to reflect on where the survivors are currently, but invites them to go beyond where they are and reflect on ways of coping with their traumatic experiences, both in terms of the interventions they have received and other ways they have used to cope. The chapter examines the interventions received by the South Sudanese participants to cope with traumatic experiences, as well as the resilience portrayed.

Chapter 6 offers a vantage point from where we, and the participants, can have an opportunity to consider the journey past and the journey ahead, and the options of how to proceed from this point forward. The chapter discusses the participants' definitions of peace and explores possibilities of peace and peacebuilding that exist in the participants' perceptions of peace, experiences of trauma, interventions received and resilience shown. Based on these perceptions and experiences, the chapter discusses what the journey towards sustainable peace may involve.

Finally, Chap. 7, the conclusion ties all the pieces of the journey together to form one whole, and derive lessons for future journeys.

The overall aim of this book is to explore the link between interventions for survivors of trauma and peacebuilding processes in conflict situations, with specific reference to South Sudanese refugees in Kakuma Refugee Camp in Kenya. This aim arises from recognizing that building sustainable peace not only needs to involve international and national efforts at the macro institutional level, but also be sensitive to the trauma of the survivors of conflict and mass violence at the individual and community level. At the background of this argument is the postulation that 'the pervasive presence of such a large segment of traumatized members at all levels of these societies poses perhaps the most formidable barrier to peace' (Olweean and Friedman 1999). The book examines how an understanding of the trauma experienced by the survivors of conflict and provision of interventions that are sensitive to these traumatic experiences, is essential in building sustainable peace.

References

Denscombe, M. (2003). *The Good Research Guide.* 2nd Edition. Maidenhed: Open University Press.

Denzin, N.K. (1989). 'The Interpretive Point of View'. In Denzin, N.K. *Interpretive Interactionism.* Newbury Park, California: Sage Publications, pp. 10–34.

Frank, A.W. (1995). *The Wounded Storyteller: Body, Illness, and Ethics*. Chicago: University of Chicago Press.

Frank, A.W. (2010). *Letting Stories Breathe.* Chicago: University of Chicago Press.

Galletta, A. (2013). *Mastering the Semi-structured Interview and Beyond; From Research Design to Analysis and Publication*. New York: New York University Press.

Olweean, S. & Friedman, S. (1999) 'Relief Project and International Peace Conference'. Common Bond Institute. Retrieved 8 July 2015 from: http://www.minelres.lv/minelres/archive/07241999-11_22_44-17900.html.

Smith, J.A. & Osborn, M. (2003). 'Interpretative phenomenological analysis'. In J.A. Smith (Ed.), *Qualitative Psychology: A Practical Guide to Research Methods.* London: Sage Publications.

Chapter 1
Understanding South Sudanese Refugees

> *The action most worth watching is not at the center of things but where edges meet... and often, if you stand at the point of tangency, you can see both sides better than if you were in the middle of either one.*
> Anne Fadiman, *The Spirit Catches You and You Fall Down*, 1997, p. viii.

1.1 The Edge of the River

Talia woke up with a mumbled scream on her lips and a sweat. She had been dreaming of the horrors she had witnessed in the hands of her captors once again. In this dream, Talia was running as fast as her legs could carry her across the plain, towards the river which she would cross into safety. The ground was thorny and the bristles on the bushes were sharp, pricking her unkindly as she ran. Her feet were worn and her thin shoes would wear out fast, she knew. Talia glanced back and saw one lone man pursuing her. The others from her family and her village had scattered in different directions when the enemies from a neighboring tribe had struck and burnt down their houses and killed her husband among others.

Her pursuer was gaining speed on her. Talia saw that he held some sort of weapon, ready to strike. She managed to reach the edge of the river which she would cross and be on safe ground where he would not pursue her any more. Where no one would pursue her. Where she would be at peace. She tried to beckon the safety boat that was carrying others across, but she could not be seen. She tried calling out but could not be heard. She realized no voice could come out of her lips. The pursuer was gaining speed towards her. She tried once more to shout for help. She woke abruptly, heart racing, her whole body soaked in sweat...

Peace, as in Talia's dream, has eluded the people of South Sudan for over five decades of civil war and the North-South conflict. The conflict in Sudan and South Sudan has gained notoriety for being the longest violent conflict in Africa, and for the effects it has had on the civilian populations, including death, disease and

L.W. Gitau, *Trauma-Sensitivity and Peacebuilding*, The Anthropocene: Politik—Economics—Society—Science 12, DOI 10.1007/978-3-319-49803-4_1

displacement. The conflict comprises two civil wars, and has a long and complex history of neglect, exclusion and marginalization of the south, dating back to pre-colonial rule (LeRiche/Arnold 2012).

This First Civil War between the Arab/Muslim North and the African/Christian South, which took place from 1955 to 1972, was led by a group of insurgents known as the *Anya-Nya.*[1] They resisted the aggressive assimilation programs of 'Arabization' and 'Islamization' of the South, and demanded Southern independence as the only solution to the problem of marginalization and exclusion of the South by the North (LeRiche/Arnold 2012). The war ended in 1972 with the Addis Ababa Agreement, which granted Southern Sudan semi-autonomy through a regional government with a representative assembly, and created constitutional provisions for religious and cultural protection. The Addis Ababa Agreement, however, did not last due to the inability of Southern Sudanese to unite politically in its defense, and the failure of the Khartoum regime of Jaafar Mohammad an-Numeiry, to meet its provisions (LeRiche/Arnold 2012; Malwal 2015).

The Second Civil War began in 1983, led by the Sudan People's Liberation Army (SPLA) with John Garang de Mabior as the leader.[2] Revolution, rather than secession, was the goal. It aimed to end the perpetuation of the idea of Sudan as an Arab-Islamic state. This war ended on 9 January 2005 with the signing of the Comprehensive Peace Agreement (CPA) in Naivasha, Kenya, between the Khartoum-based regime of Omar Hassan al-Bashir and his National Congress Party (NCP) and the Sudan People's Liberation Army/Movement (SPLA/M). The war lasted 22 years and is estimated to have killed two million people and rendered another four million homeless (LeRiche/Arnold 2012).

Reflecting on the signing of the CPA, Atem, one of the participants in the research said:

> *Though the CPA was signed in 2005, there was still insecurity in South Sudan. The government had not reinforced and sustained security for the people. And we the Sudanese are very good in revenging. We want to avenge the blood of our brothers and sisters who have been killed.*[3]

---

[1]*Anya-Nya* means 'snake venom' in Madi Language, spoken in parts of Uganda and South Sudan. The *Anya-Nya* were a group of separatists led by Joseph Lagu, and formed the military wing of the Southern Sudan Resistance Movement (SSRM). They fought the First Sudanese Civil War, or Anya Nya Rebellion, from 1963 until 1972, when Lagu and the Sudanese president, Jaafar Muhammad an-Numeiry, signed the Addis Ababa Agreement (Boddy-Evans n.d.).

[2]John Garang led the Sudan People's Liberation Army (SPLA) and served as the first Vice President of Sudan from 9 July 2005 until his death in a plane crash on 30 July 2005. He is considered very influential in the politics of South Sudan, especially amongst the Dinka people of South Sudan.

[3]Interview with Atem (not his real name) on 2 July 2013. See Appendix 1.1. All the participants of the research were given pseudonyms.

The signing of the CPA ushered in the six-year Interim Period which was premised upon making unity attractive for the Sudan. It allowed South Sudan a referendum on full independence after the six-year period. South Sudan's independence was seen as a possibility, but unity was to be attempted. This failed in its purpose and culminated in an almost unanimous vote for independence by Southern Sudanese in a referendum held in January 2011. The CPA also addressed the conflict in Southern Kordofan, near the border of Sudan and South Sudan, giving the people some measure of autonomy that would give them a right to have their views sought on their system of governance through popular consultation.

On 9 July 2011, South Sudan seceded from the larger Sudan and the new Republic of South Sudan was born. This was fifty-five years after Sudan's own independence from British rule on 1 January 1956. As LeRiche/Arnold (2012: ix)

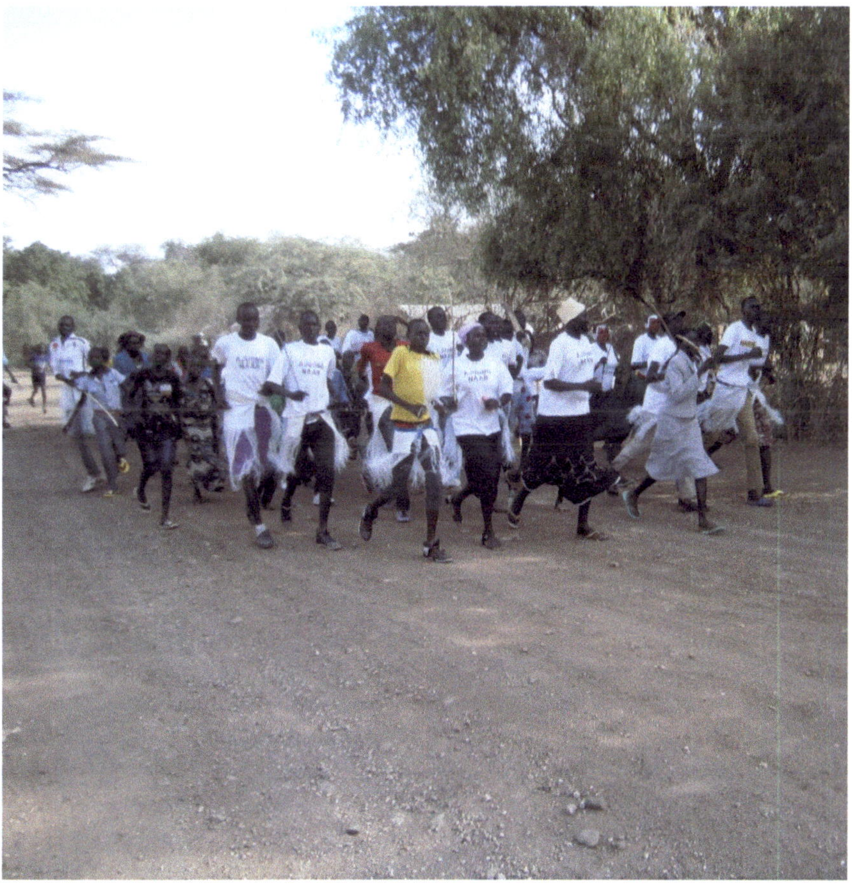

South Sudanese refugees in Kakuma commemorate South Sudan Independence Day with a tribal dance. *Source* The Author

point out, achieving internal peace posed a major challenge, and resolving the persistent issues of 'oppressive governance, exploitation, and marginalization', would be critical to South Sudan's success or failure as a state, since gaining independence is not synonymous with achieving peace. Further, the challenge of reconciliation among the tribes of South Sudan, and the need for the South Sudanese people to build an identity based on harmony rather than a collective opposition to the North, would be of interest to the new nation. The outcome of the secession has however been undesirable on several fronts. Sorbo/Ahmed (2013: 1) note that

> The reality soon came to look quite different. South Sudan celebrated its independence before the terms of divorce had been agreed upon. A number of issues remained unresolved, including disputed borders, citizenship issues, fees for shipping southern oil through northern pipelines, and the future status of Abyei area on the border. There was also the problem of the aborted popular consultations in South Kordofan and Blue Nile States. In June 2011, a new war started in the Nuba Mountains in South Kordofan.

This new war in the Nuba Mountains in South Kordofan is of particular importance as it indicated the complex and often intertwined realities facing both Sudan and South Sudan post-secession, especially at the borderlands.

The political disputes related to land dispossession, competition for resources, economic, social and political marginalization easily and quickly spiral into ethnic targeting and communal mobilization, as different ethnic groups scramble for the available resources as well as political recognition and influence to counter their feelings of marginalization. Cattle rustling among the agropastoralist tribes of the Dinka, Nuer and Murle for instance, as they compete for economic resources, is a particularly common source of conflict, violence and displacement.

Renewed fighting erupted between rival units of the Sudan People's Liberation Army (SPLA) in Juba on 15 December 2013. According to International Crisis Group (2014), this fighting displaced more than one million people and killed more than 10,000. The rival parties, predominantly represented by Dinka constituents associated with the South Sudanese President, Salva Kirr, and Nuer constituents associated with the former Vice President, Riek Machar on opposing sides, engaged in systematic violence targeted against each other and mostly leading to civilian casualties. An Integrated Regional Information Networks (IRIN) report (2014) notes that this renewed violence was 'in fact the culmination of a long-simmering power struggle between different people and groups within the ruling Sudan People's Liberation Movement/Army' that was less apparent during decades of the North-South conflict. The international community's intervention and the regional Intergovernmental Authority on Development's (IGAD) attempts at brokering peace between the warring South Sudan parties in Addis Ababa, Ethiopia (CEWARN 2014), have not born much fruit, and peace remains distant for the South Sudanese.

Talia vaguely remembered that she had heard that some people, big people, John Garang[4] *or Salva Kiir and Riek Machar and others she did not know, were meeting in some far away country to talk about peace. She did not know what they were talking about. She only wanted her disturbing dreams to stop. And to live again.*

When Talia slept that following night, she dreamt again. The same dream. Her pursuer was close by now. Should she jump into the crocodile-infested river to escape him, she wondered. She stood immobilized and waited in resignation. She glanced at him. He seemed so small when he was close by. Like a young boy, the age of her son. Was this her pursuer? She looked him over as he slowed down. He did not strike. He was carrying a large stick, not a spear! She looked at his eyes. There were tears there, and a fear. She glanced at his feet. They were bleeding! He had no shoes, and had been running after her on the thorns and bristles until his feet were badly wounded. Now he just stood there, silent. She reached to her feet and took off her shoes and gave them to him. He took them. Talia understood.

This book is cognizant of the nuanced ways in which the South Sudanese refugees experienced the war back in South Sudan and its consequences, their disparate journeys in search of refuge, their diverse experiences of the interventions they receive in Kakuma refugee camp and their perceptions of peace. Importantly, this book acknowledges the fading nature of boundaries surrounding categorizations when they are placed around people's experiences and perceptions of events such as war. Just as Talia could no longer recognize her pursuer as her enemy in the end, but rather identified with him as a victim too, we find the interplay of the experiences, perceptions and the relationships in the South Sudanese conflict is complex. This book does not lay claim to the answer to the puzzle why peace is elusive to South Sudan, but seeks to illuminate a part of the puzzle by inviting us to 'the edge of the river', to watch and participate in what happens in an attempt to understand how we might get to the other side of the river, the side of peace.

As a result of the recurrent instability and threats to security, many South Sudanese civilians have fled their country to seek refuge in camps in neighbouring countries. Kakuma Refugee Camp in Kenya has been a key destination for many of the fleeing South Sudanese through the years of conflict and violence, including those fleeing conflict and violencein the emerging 'new South' at the borderlands such as South Kordofan. They arrive in Kakuma fleeing attack, having lost all possessions and having witnessed their family members killed or separated from them. These refugees, survivors of the conflict and mass violence in their homeland, are central to the themes explored in this book.

[4]Though John Garang died on 30 July 2005, after the signing of the Comprehensive Peace Agreement (CPA) on 9 July 2005, Talia in this description refers to him as though he is still alive. This reference indicates the remoteness of the peace talks in the perception of the civilians who bear the brunt of the violence in South Sudan.

1.2 Kakuma Refugee Camp

Kakuma Refugee Camp lies in the semi-arid Turkana District of the Northwestern region of Kenya, East Africa. It houses about 180,000 refugees who have fled war from neighbouring countries, mainly South Sudan, Somalia, Ethiopia, Eritrea, Burundi and the Democratic Republic of Congo (DRC), with 91,474 of the refugees being from South Sudan, as of June 2015 (UNHCR 2015a).

The camp lies about 100 km south of the South Sudan-Kenya border, and approximately 1000 km from Nairobi (Horn 2010). It was established in 1992 to serve as a temporary refuge for about 20,000 unaccompanied minors from Sudan (popularly known as 'The Lost Boys')[5] (UNICEF 1996). For a number of refugees, the camp has become a long-term destination and the only home they practically know of. The refugees co-exist with local nomadic Turkana people, whose lifestyle is focused on livestock and live in an extremely harsh environment.

Most of the South Sudanese refugees in Kakuma are not able to return to their country of origin for reasons ranging from recurring violence to political insecurity. Many of the refugees hope to be resettled in one of the few countries that receive refugees, which include United States of America, Australia, Canada and Scandinavian countries. However, only a very limited number (less than 5%) of those awaiting resettlement are resettled due to the overwhelming number of resettlement needs, the limited number of countries that receive resettlement cases, and the limited capacity of UNHCR to process resettlement cases (UNHCR 2014).

The camp is administered by the UNHCR, which depends on donations from the international community to meet its budget. To provide services to the refugees, UNHCR works with its implementing partners which include the World Food Programme (WFP), International Organization for Migration (IOM), the Kenya Red Cross Society, Lutheran World Federation (LWF), Norwegian Refugee Council (NRC), Refugee Consortium of Kenya, Don Bosco—Kenya, FilmAid International, Jesuit Refugee Services (JRS), International Rescue Committee (IRC), National Council of Churches of Kenya (NCCK), and Windle Trust Kenya (WTK) (UNHCR 2015b).

The refugees depend almost entirely on these agencies to meet their basic needs. Due to the harsh, semi-arid climate of Northwestern Kenya where the camp is located, the refugees are not able to grow any crops in the camp. Further, they are not allowed to keep any animals, neither are they allowed to seek formal employment (Horn 2010). UNHCR and the partnering organizations provide jobs for about 2000 refugees who are paid 'incentives', not salaries, of about 4000 Kenya Shillings (40 USD) per month. A number of refugees engage in trade and commercial activities within the camp, which include selling food items, clothing

[5]A discussion of 'The Lost Boys', some of whom are refugees in Kakuma and were interviewed, appears in Chap. 4 in relation to the issue of identity (Powell 2015).

and other household wares, and providing communication services. A few South Sudanese operate as petty traders, but most businesses are operated by Somali and Ethiopian refugees (Eisei 2014: 224).

1.3 Conclusion

The experiences of the South Sudanese refugees are varied and complex. Many are attacked in their country of origin and witness family members and neighbours being killed. Those who survive the killing disperse and families are separated as each person flees their own way, escaping the attack. They walk for long distances seeking refuge, with no rest and little or no food or water. Some are eventually able to get transport means by lorry or plane to reach the South Sudan/Kenya border, while others walk the whole way. On the way they face insecurity, hunger and thirst, and constantly worry about loved ones who were killed and others whose whereabouts they do not know.

They are eventually ferried to Kakuma from the border, and received at the Reception Centre. They are registered as refugees in the camp by UNHCR, given a ration card that allows them identification as refugees, and enables them to access food, shelter, health and education facilities. They wait at the reception centre for about a month and are resettled in the community in the camp. They are given housing materials to construct their own houses.

Within the community in the camp they continue to receive the services of a food ration and health facilities, and many of them go to school in the camp. Some get employment with the agencies that work in the camp in partnership with UNHCR. Some look for other ways of survival, and start small businesses to augment the supplies they get from UNHCR. As they settle in the camp, many remember and are disturbed by the events they experienced back in their country of origin, especially the separation from, and death of, loved ones. They suffer loneliness and a sense of insecurity and uncertainty about their future. Some receive counselling for their stress, and many turn to the education opportunities in the camp to cope, immersing themselves in these opportunities. Some turn to leadership opportunities in the camp, focusing more on serving others in the community.

The survivors face disease, and even death in the camp. Cultural practices such as paying dowry for a bride, differing gender roles and wife inheritance after one's husband dies are affected by the new setting in the camp. Many turn to faith or religion as a source of solace. Others look to resettlement in a developed country as the solution to their troubles.

Some of the survivors are hopeful for peace in their lives and in their country of origin, and see their role in helping achieve this peace through involvement in the community and through education. To others, peace in their lives and in their country of origin seems far-fetched and they neither relate to it, believe in it, nor see how they can contribute to achieving it.

Appendix 1.1

Pseudonym	M/F	Ethnic group	Age	Duration of stay in the camp	Brief details	Date of interview
Atem	M	Dinka	42	21 years	Community leader. Married, with four children. Had gone back to South Sudan in 1999 to participate in the war and came back to the camp in 2005. Incentive worker with IRC. Was among 'The Lost Boys'	2 July 2013

References

Boddy-Evans, A. (n.d) 'Anya-nya'. Retrieved 18 July 2015 from: http://africanhistory.about.com/od/glossarya2/g/Anya-Nya.htm.

Conflict Early Warning and Response (2014). 'Peace Talks on South Sudan'.

Eisei, K. (2014). 'Changing Identifications among the Pari Refugees in Kakuma'. In Schlee, G. & Watson, E.E. (Eds.) *Changing Identification and Alliances in North-East Africa. Vol. II: Sudan, Uganda and Ethiopia-Sudan Borderlands*. New York: Berghahn, pp. 223–233.

Horn, R. (2010). 'Exploring the Impact of Displacement and Encampment on Domestic Violence in Kakuma Refugee Camp'. In *Journal of Refugee Studies* Vol. 23, No. 3, pp. 356–376.

International Crisis Group (2014). 'Conflict Alert: Halting South Sudan's Spreading Civil War'. Retrieved 19 March 2015 from: http://www.responsibilitytoprotect.org/index.php/crises/196-crisis-in-south-sudan/5479-international-crisis-group-conflict-alert-halting-south-sudans-spreading-civil-war.

International Regional Information Networks (2014). 'How did we get here?' Retrieved 19 March 2015 from: https://www.irinnews.org/film/4980/south-sudan-how-did-we-get-here.

LeRiche, M. & Arnold, M. (2012). *South Sudan: From Revolution to Independence*. London: Hurst & Company.

Malwal, B. (2015). *Sudan and South Sudan: From One to Two*. Hampshire: Palgrave Macmillan.

Sorbo, G.M. & Ahmed, G. M. (2013). 'Introduction: Sudan's Durable Disorder'. In Sorbo, G.M and Ahmed, A.G. (Eds.) *Sudan Divided: Continuing conflict in a Contested State*. New York: Palgrave Macmillan, pp. 1–24.

UNHCR (2014). 'UNHCR Projected Global Resettlement Needs'. Retrieved 21 January 2016 from: http://www.unhcr.org/51e3eabf9.html.

UNHCR (2015a). 'Figures at a Glance'. Retrieved on 28 May 2015 from: http://www.unhcr.org/pages/49c3646c11.html.
UNHCR (2015b). '2015 UNHCR Country Operations Profile—Kenya'. Retrieved 20 January 2016 from: http://www.unhcr.org/pages/49e483a16.html.
UNICEF (1996). 'The Lost Boys of the Sudan'. Retrieved 9 May 2015 from: http://www.unicef.org/sowc96/closboys.htm.

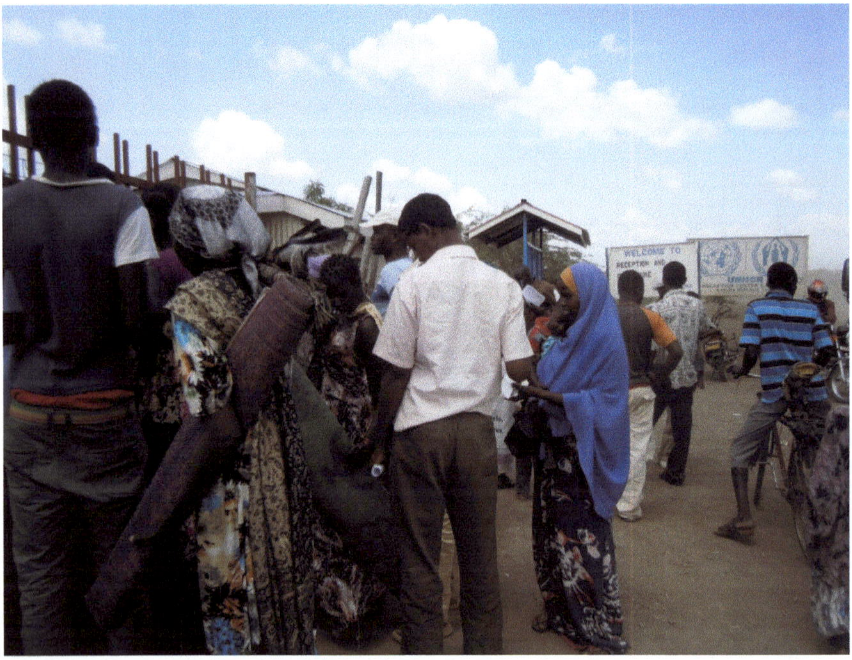

Newly arrived refugees at the Kakuma Refugee Camp Reception Centre. *Source* The Author

Chapter 2
The Trauma-Sensitivity Gap

2.1 No Peace for Grace

> *I came to Kakuma in 1999 because of the Sudan war. We had to flee for our lives. My brother was accused of treason, of having joined a rebel group, was captured and was killed. They then captured my father, tied a dog to his back, beat the dog, and the dog mauled my father to death. Now I am here in Kakuma. I live with the children of my brother, 10 children. Plus one child of mine. I've given birth to 14 children, 13 have died and only one has survived.*
>
> *Back in South Sudan, I had a husband who held me by force (raped me), as a result of the war. I lived with him as his wife, we had children, but they could not survive, as a result of the war. Now I can't go back there...*
>
> *There is no peace for me in South Sudan at all. Other people may have peace, but there is no peace for me... But I really wish I could find a way to have peace in my heart and my body.*[1]

This was part of Grace's story as she related the experiences that led to her fleeing for refuge in Kakuma. The emotional, the physical and the external for her tend to merge and determine her experience of peace or lack thereof.

There is a growing acknowledgement that the experiences of trauma that the survivors of conflict and mass violence go through during, and after, the conflict need to be addressed, for peace to be sustainable. This acknowledgement is born out of a recognition that peacebuilding specifically focused on the national realm, attempted through international intervention and that seeks to strengthen national institutions, has not been very successful in achieving sustainable peace (Samuels 2005: 663–664).

The Catastrophic Trauma Recovery (CTR) project (Common Bond Institute 2014) identifies psychological and emotional injuries as 'the most enduring effects

[1]Interview with Grace on 17th July 2013. See Appendix 2.1.

L.W. Gitau, *Trauma-Sensitivity and Peacebuilding*, The Anthropocene: Politik—Economics—Society—Science 12, DOI 10.1007/978-3-319-49803-4_2

of war, yet historically the least addressed in terms of rebuilding a society and preventing future violence'. According to the project, significant recovery efforts usually focus on more visible needs such as food, shelter, clothing, physical health, and economic aid, and overlook or minimize the effects of deep psychological trauma on individuals, their families, and their communities. Trauma becomes embedded as part of the psyche of a society that extends the wounds into future generations where it is often played out in further violence (Volkan 2001; Lambourne/Niyonzima 2015). The cycle of violence and the cycle of trauma thus directly contribute to each other.

Strengthening of national institutions, supporting democracy, improving public services and encouraging attempts at reconciliation are all important interventions in conflict and post conflict situations. However, they are not sufficient in and of themselves. There is need to engage the survivors in ways that address their psychological, spiritual, emotional, and physical needs (LeBaron 2003). This kind of approach allows for practices that keep the survivors, like Grace, ready to navigate the change and confusion that often accompany encounters in conflict and post-conflict societies. It considers at its core the rebuilding of individuals and communities.

Judging from the conflicts, massacres and wars in South Sudan which have been mostly intra-state, it appears that current strategies for dealing with conflict need to be augmented. There has therefore been a need for a shift in the character of analyses and response to these conflicts. Traditional approaches to diplomacy and peacebuilding which typically viewed the nation-state as the sole or fundamental unit in international relations have needed to change to approaches that are more community and individual-based (Dress 2005).

The failure of contemporary peace processes to result to sustainable peace may be attributed to the failure to address the bitterness, memories and images associated with the conflict and mass violence. This points to the need for the participation of the survivors in peacebuilding work or what Gawerc (2006: 445) calls 'grassroots peace work' and 'people-to-people activities', an area she argues is plagued by limited academic research.

The failure to address the pain and traumas of the survivors of conflict and mass violence has a subtle but grievous effect on peacebuilding. The traumas may affect the social functioning of individuals and ability to support themselves and their families. Further, exposure to traumatic events and high levels of mental distress may also influence respondent attitudes to reconciliation. Patrick, one of the participants in the research, had been a livestock health professional back in South Sudan before being displaced, and had worked directly in communities educating them in peace and conflict management. Now as a refugee in Kakuma, he found himself in a precarious situation, not able to be of much help, and says:

> *We had a lot of difficulties getting to Kakuma from South Sudan. All the money we had got finished, and the children were very vulnerable and almost died of starvation. When we got to the Reception Centre, we faced more difficulties before we got registered and were given*

the ration card. ... At the Reception Centre they used to bring some kind of music, to promote healing, and also some videos, informally. I don't think it helped though, because people were still fighting even at the Reception Centre, since they were traumatized. I think the psychosocial activities were not sufficient...Because our people are traumatized. I'm also traumatized, because we are affected by the war, by seeing people being killed.[2]

Decreased interest or participation in important activities, feeling disconnected from others, a sense of no hope for the future, and a sense of despondency that leads to neglect of personal and professional responsibilities may render the survivors of conflict-inflicted trauma unable to engage in meaningful peacebuilding activities (Gasana 2008). The community's social order may be eroded, and its ability to care for its vulnerable people through, for instance, community self-support can be affected. Social cohesion can diminish as individuals withdraw, preoccupied with their own traumatic experience, resulting in disharmony and possibility of recurring violence (Gutlove/Thompson 2006). These arguments about the disruption of social cohesion linked to the effects of unaddressed trauma could help explain how quickly South Sudan erupted into civil war along ethnic lines barely two years after its independence from the Sudan. Addressing these problems with a sensitivity to the trauma the survivors have experienced, thus becomes crucial.

2.2 A Shift to Mental Health and Psychosocial Support in Peacebuilding

With the acknowledgement of the inadequacy of peacebuilding aimed at strengthening national institutions as discussed, and the recognition of the impact of mass violence on the mental and social health of the survivors, the shift of the character of analyses and response to conflict and mass violence has indeed taken place. This shift is particularly notable through the growing field of Mental Health and Psychosocial Support (MHPSS). In 2007 the Inter-Agency Standing Committee (IASC) established by the United Nations General Assembly to coordinate, develop policies and make decisions on the work of key humanitarian agencies, formulated guidelines on 'Mental Health and Psychosocial Support (MHPSS) in Emergency Settings' to enable effective coordination of the work of mental health practitioners and psychosocial support workers in the context of emergencies arising from armed conflict and natural disasters (IASC 2007). These guidelines are based on the acknowledgement of the psychological and social impacts of emergencies on the mental health and psychosocial well-being of those affected, as discussed above, and the potential threat of this impact on peace, human rights and development (IASC 2007: 1).

The term 'mental health and psychosocial support' refers to 'any type of local or outside support that aims to protect or promote psychosocial well-being and/or

[2] Interview with Patrick on 15th and 16th July 2013. See Appendix 2.1.

prevent or treat mental disorder (IASC 2007: 1). Psychosocial support refers to interventions that address the psychological aspects of experience, such as feelings and emotions, and the social aspects of experience, such as relationships and culture (Hamber et al. 2014: 8). While these guidelines are established on firm principles of upholding and protecting the human rights of the affected populations, recognising and building on their capacities, and respecting the intertwined and complex nature of the interventions (IASC 2007: 9–13) the IASC noted the limited research base and need for more evidence for what interventions, under MHPSS, would be most effective (IASC 2007: 2). Commenting on this need for more research in the MHPSS field, Hamber et al. (2014) note that

> … attempts to build an evidence base for MHPSS have focused on clinical MHPSS services (by mental health specialists and psychotherapists)… Relatively limited attention has been given to the effects of broad community based psychosocial interventions on collective wellbeing and social connectedness. We believe this is an important issue that needs to be addressed… More specifically, can and do psychosocial interventions and practices shape long-term collective social processes of peacebuilding and wider social change, including processes such as development and social transformation? (Hamber et al. 2014: 8).

The exploration of trauma interventions, which fall under the broad category of psychosocial interventions for survivors of conflict and mass violence in this book, addresses this concern in part.

In May 2015, the Institute for Justice and Reconciliation(IJR) (South Africa) and the War Trauma Foundation (WTF) (Netherlands) hosted a conference in Johannesburg, South Africa, to address the nexus and linkage between the fields of peacebuilding and mental health and psychosocial services (MHPSS), noting that ‘While both fields contribute vital services to affected communities, their work takes place largely in isolation of the other’ (IJR 2015). The IJR noted in particular that there are only a few studies that explicitly link psychosocial work and peacebuilding, and there was need for research to inform the understanding of what MHPSS interventions influence processes of building sustainable peace. The following section discusses a cross-section of the studies that have addressed this link within the last 16 years, and identifies where this book comes in, in contributing to this link.

In 1999, Woodside and colleagues published a study on ‘Psychological Trauma and Social Healing in Croatia’, discussing their project which was aimed at promoting trauma healing, non-violent conflict resolution, peaceful living, human rights, and reduction of ethnic bias in Croatian children affected by war. The study was based on the premise that ‘psychological healing and social healing were interdependent and mutually reinforcing (Woodside et al. 1999: 355). The outcome of the intervention indicated significant reduction of post-traumatic symptoms and ethnic bias, and increased acceptance of non-violent conflict resolution methods and girls’ self-esteem (Woodside et al. 1999: 363). This outcome indicates a direct link between psychosocial work and peacebuilding.

Hart/Colo’s (2014) study on ‘Psychosocial peacebuilding in Bosnia and Herzegovina’ is another example of works explicitly linking psychosocial work and peacebuilding in the Balkans. Hart/Colo (2014) present two projects carried out in post war Bosnia and Herzegovina, the first one by CARE International through its Welcome and Information Project (WICP) in 1996, and the second one by Catholic Relief Services (CRS) through its Choosing Peace Together (CPT) project, 15 years later. The two projects aimed to examine and address the psychological and social impact of the traumatic events the survivors were exposed to. The projects involved educating the survivors on psychosocial trauma and creating safe spaces for them to tell their stories. The healing processes included storytelling, listening, building trust and transforming relationships between individuals, groups and communities. According to Hart/Colo's (2014: 80) report, the projects were instrumental in transforming the conflict 'relationally, economically and politically'. Of particular note is the theories of change that informed the work (Hart/Colo: 82). These included an assumption that if people could overcome their trauma, build trust and change relationships, this could lead to the formation of new narratives, which would lead to peace between groups who were originally in conflict. The other theory of change held that if people involved in the project could share their experiences with other members, these other members would be open to contact with people they had previously demonized, and this could lead to trust and confidence between groups. This attention to the theories of change in application in these projects points to the need for explicit connection of psychosocial work and peacebuilding in the very design of the projects, to make outcomes more tangible.

A similar clarity of the theoretical base for psychosocial work and peacebuilding can be noted in Lykes' (2000) study. Lykes discusses the contribution of liberation psychology in designing and implementing interventions geared towards transforming conflict and building peace amongst communities affected by mass violence. Liberation psychology, an approach of psychology articulated by Martín-Baró (1994) seeks to understand the psychology of the oppressed and the poor, and with this understanding help to address the oppressive structures and liberate the people from the effects of their experiences under these structures. Lykes used participatory action research (PAR) among Mayan women of rural Guatemala, whereby the women used photography as a resource for constructing and telling the stories of their experiences of the war, how it had affected them, and their responses to the war (Lykes 2000: 384). Lykes notes that the project facilitated the building of trust and confidence amongst participants, as well as envisioning possibilities for moving forward after the war (Lykes 2000: 391).

Fuertes' (2004) work facilitating community trauma healing workshops amongst Karen Refugees in a refugee camp along the Thailand-Burmese border in 2003 offers another example of studies directly connecting psychosocial support and peacebuilding. Fuertes argues:

> … when people are traumatized in terms of having been enveloped by deep-seated pain, hurt, frustration, and disappointment to the extent of becoming angry and vengeful or withdrawn from social and public life, no amount of peace talks or agreements can rebuild their community and mend shattered relationships (Fuertes 2004: 492).

Fuertes advocates for the integration of trauma healing in the peacebuilding processes, and further underscores the need to hear the survivors voices regarding their sense of reality and ways of coping through conducting studies on war-induced traumas or what he calls 'warviews', and how these views impact on survivors' coping mechanisms (Fuertes 2004: 492). This book seeks to contribute in part to this need through attention to the voices of the South Sudanese refugees in Kakuma.

In addition to the need to listen to the voices of the survivors, a need for a framework in establishing the link has been noted. Silove (2004) proposes a framework to reconcile mental health initiatives with the overall mission of humanitarian services for communities affected by conflict and mass violence, based on his experience in post-conflict East Timor. His proposed framework generally encourages survival and adaptation of individuals and communities in the contexts of mass violence, and specifically reinforces systems of adaptation that include 'the re-establishment of safety and security, the restoration of interpersonal bonds, the creation of systems of justice, the development of a social framework that allows survivors to develop new roles and identities, and the revival of institutions that confer meaning' (Silove 2004: 93). Such a framework attempts to link the psychological, the social and the political.

This link between the psychological, the social and the political in the context of conflict and mass violence is further alluded to by Ramanathapillai in his article 'The Politicizing of Trauma: A Case Study of Sri Lanka' (2006). Ramanathapillai problematizes storytelling and argues that the same narratives of pain and suffering that are used for healing trauma, can sometimes be exploited by violent factions amongst the affected populations to promote aggression, as in the case of Tamil nationalists and militants in Sri Lanka. This occurs through selectively choosing and emphasising certain aspects of the traumatic event while omitting others when relating the experiences, and thus influencing the collective understanding of the event. In this way, the stories 'serve as tools to create conformity of vision and purpose and perpetuate a cultural and political identity of victimhood' (Ramanathapillai 2006: 5). Ramanathapillai concludes that this politicising of trauma results in perpetuating the cycle of trauma amongst the Tamils, and calls for the merging of mental health and education initiatives with peacebuilding as part of 'creative and imaginative initiatives' needed to heal the wounds of war (Ramanathapillai 2006: 16).

In his conceptualization of the 'Peacebuilding Wheel', Hart (2008: viii–ix), Hart/Colo's (2014) directly links psychosocial work and peacebuilding, underscoring the importance of trauma-sensitivity in peacebuilding which consists of '*tangible*' and '*intangible*' elements forming the various spokes of the wheel. Tangible elements include the objectified, measurable issues such as reconstruction of infrastructure, peace agreements, political arrangements, and humanitarian assistance in basic necessities such as food, shelter and health facilities. The intangible elements are less measurable and include psychological issues such as the experience of trauma, stress, threat of identity loss, and spiritual needs. As Hart/Colo's (2014) further points out, the tangible and intangible issues are intertwined in their role in peacebuilding, and act synergetically to enhance a more sustainable peacebuilding process. Each spoke of the wheel is important, and the absence of any may cause the imbalance and eventual toppling of the wheel. Importantly, a trauma-sensitivity is necessary in attending to even the tangible elements of the peacebuilding wheel, for peace to be sustainable. Hart argues:

> ...if the more tangible issues are not seen to have psychological or symbolic importance in the reconstruction phase after war, this, too, may contribute to ineffective approaches to rebuilding communities and societies after large-scale violence and war (Hart 2008: viii).

Gallagher et al. (2012) in their work 'Perspectives and Possibilities: Mental Health in post-Agreement Northern Ireland', similarly point to this link. They question the efficacy of conceptualising mental health problems in the context of post-conflict reconstruction 'as a definable and diagnosable psychopathology' rather than a wider social problem (Gallagher et al. 2012: 63). Recognising the pervasive impact of conflict on the mental health and the social health of survivors, Gallagher and her colleagues advocate for stretching of the boundaries of the mental health field to include the areas of politics, justice, socio-economics and education, and envision well-integrated community-oriented interventions with 'psychological, social, economic, cultural and environmental elements' (Gallagher et al. 2012: 71). Clancy/Hamber (2008: 9) point to this intertwined relationship of the social and the mental health areas in conceptualizing trauma healing in the context of complex political emergencies when they point out that 'What needs to be "healed" is therefore the multitude of individual, political, social, and cultural responses to a traumatic situation and its aftermath.' Clancy/Hamber (2008: 38) thus argue that addressing trauma after mass violence needs to be placed in the wider context of peacebuilding and development initiatives, and reciprocally, peacebuilding needs to be encompassed in trauma healing programs.

In the same vein, Pupavac (2004: 491) points out the need to look beyond epidemiological literature to understand trauma and its effects in contexts of mass violence, and argues that psychosocial work as part of humanitarian intervention is not apolitical, thus indirectly pointing to the interrelatedness of psychosocial support and peacebuilding. If we see conflict, which results in exposure to traumatic events for the survivors, as a political affair, then in addressing the trauma and engaging in peacebuilding as a response to the conflict, we are engaging in a political affair, as much as a social and psychological one.

This link is further identified by Lambourne/Gitau (2013) in their study on the role of psychosocial interventions in peacebuilding and development in Rwanda after the 1994 genocide. Lambourne and Gitau argue that psychosocial interventions contribute to a holistic and transformative approach to peacebuilding, shifting from a focus on 'the top-down, state-driven peacebuilding efforts that seek to strengthen national institutions and service provision but fail to promote an emancipatory, sustainable or transformative peace' (p. 33). Lambourne and Gitau conclude that an integration of trauma healing and other psychosocial services into the national and international peacebuilding efforts could result in more sustainable peace and development.

A key issue in the studies linking psychosocial support and peacebuilding has been the question of how relevant the interventions are to the affected population. With this regard, Eiling and colleagues (2014) carried out research amongst children in the Eastern Equatoria State of South Sudan, using War Child Holland's psychosocial support intervention I DEAL, which is aimed at improving the coping ability of children and young people affected by conflict and mass violence. The research sought to assess whether I DEAL was an appropriate and relevant intervention for the young people in South Sudan, as well as seeking to strengthen the evidence base on the effectiveness of psychosocial interventions for children and young people (Eiling et al. 2014: 63). I DEAL addressed the themes of identity, emotions, relationships with peers, relationships with adults, conflict and peace, and the future (Eiling et al. 2014: 62). These authors found I DEAL to be consistent with local perceptions of wellbeing, and as having potential for reducing violence, strengthening relationships, and thus contributing to peacebuilding processes (Eiling et al. 2014: 72). In addition, while Ameresekere/Henderson's (2012: 10) specifically focus on mental health and investigating the common psychiatrist conditions of South Sudanese in their study, they also note the need for advocacy, training and focused research to 'identify the scope of mental illness and provide culturally-meaningful interventions' for the survivors.

An overall study in the field of MHPSS was carried out by Tol and colleagues in 2011, seeking to link practices that are commonly implemented in the field, with evidence from evaluations of interventions (Tol et al. 2011). They identified counselling, community-based social supports, structured social activities, provision of information, psychosocial education, and raising awareness as the most commonly used interventions (Tol et al. 2011: 1588). One of the major findings of their study was the disconnection between research and practice, noting that there was evidence of more research focus on interventions that were less frequently used, such as a focus on PTSD. Among the recommendations Tol et al. make based on their research is the need to strengthen the evidence for MHPSS in humanitarian settings, which will involve 'a concerted effort by researchers to increase the rigour of studies and broaden outcomes beyond PTSD and internalizing symptoms' (Tol et al. 2011: 1588). They also recommend increased research focus on the more frequently used interventions such as counselling and community supports, to reduce the gap between research and practice (p. 1589). This book seeks to contribute to reducing this gap through a focus on trauma-sensitivity in peacebuilding for South Sudanese refugees.

In his examination of the intersection between trauma and peacebuilding, Zelizer (2008: 81) highlights the ethical responsibility that peacebuilding practitioners have to ensure that they are trauma-sensitive in their work, which entails, for one, desisting from categorizing the entire affected population as traumatized, secondly being careful not to cause further trauma for the survivors, and thirdly recognizing the differentiated and context-informed ways in which people respond to trauma. Similarly, the National Centre for PTSD (Post Traumatic Stress Disorder) (2011), in identifying the core issues in early intervention for trauma survivors that need to be addressed, critiques a wholesale application of psychological intervention methods and points to the need for seeking appropriate interventions based on the individuals and communities in question.

Indeed there would be many benefits of studies seeking to identify the appropriate interventions for the affected populations in question, for one, to avoid what transcultural psychiatrist Kleinman (1977: 4) termed 'a category fallacy', referring to the tendency to superimpose a diagnostic category derived in one cultural context on another culture. With this regard, De Jong (2005: 368) notes the need for studies on traumatic stress reactions from different cultures among the affected population, based on a phenomenological approach. These type of studies would inform the kind of interventions to be used in different contexts. This book seeks to add to the repertoire of such studies.

Yoder (2013: 2) likewise argues that organizations working with survivors of trauma need to be 'trauma-informed', which entails integrating a trauma-sensitive framework into any project, be it economic, health, or governance, and 'means more than putting a psychologist on every project team.' Being trauma-informed, according to Yoder (2013: 2), includes embracing a holistic outlook in considering the impact of trauma on the survivors of traumatic events, taking into account the differentiated and culturally inclined ways the affected people experience trauma beyond the traditional mental health diagnosis, and engaging diverse processes from different fields to address trauma and enhance the resilience of the affected populations.

The subject of resilience in survivors of violent conflict is crucial to a discussion of the link between psychosocial intervention and peacebuilding. Harvey (2007) makes a significant contribution in her essay discussing resilience in trauma survivors. In this study, she seeks to investigate the nature of wellness-enhancing interventions and empowering social change. She argues that this investigation can inform trauma-focused interventions at individual, community and societal levels. Pfefferbaum et al. (2008) also provide a treatise on community resilience in the face of disasters, proposing a set of contributing factors, identifying potential barriers, and making recommendations for enhancing community resilience.[3] Gallagher et al. (2012) however caution against a mistaken perception of resilience as being universally inherent in survivors of mass violence, and point to the potential danger of this perspective hindering the promotion of mental health.

[3]The concept of community resilience as it relates to the participants of this research is discussed in detail in Chap. 5.

2.3 Conclusion

A failure to attend to the traumas of the survivors of conflict and mass violence may lead to destruction of the social cohesion and social functioning of individuals and communities, decreased participation in peacebuilding activities, and psychological wounds being played out in further violence. This may explain how quickly South Sudan erupted into renewed violence, barely two years after its secession from the larger Sudan.

There has been a shift of focus to the growing field of MHPSS, as the cross-section of studies discussed has shown. These studies sought to link peacebuilding and psychosocial interventions, and show the important role that psychosocial interventions play in peacebuilding. The studies underscore the gap identified in the limited research base for what interventions should be included under MHPSS, the need for a theoretical base for the interventions, the need for the survivors' voices in identifying and implementing the interventions, the need to identify creative and imaginative initiatives, and the need for context-specific studies, based on a phenomenological approach. This book seeks to contribute to filling this gap.

Appendix 2.1

Pseudonym	M/F	Ethnic group	Age	Duration of stay in the camp	Brief details	Date of interview
Grace	F	Acholi	40	14 years	Father and brother tortured and killed on being suspected to be traitors. Raped and forced into marriage by a soldier. Has given birth 14 times and only one child has survived. Also taking care of 10 of her deceased brothers' children. Was diagnosed HIV positive in the camp and resettlement process stalled. Cooks food for sale to supplement the ration in the camp	17th July 2013

(continued)

(continued)

Pseudonym	M/F	Ethnic group	Age	Duration of stay in the camp	Brief details	Date of interview
Patrick	M	Murle	40	5 months	People from the Nuer Community attacked his village and killed many people, his wife and children ran to the bush where his wife delivered their last child. SPLA soldiers attacked his village, many people were killed and he sustained injuries. Worked as a Livestock officer. In the Reconciliation committee between the Murle and the Nuer in the camp	15th and 16th July 2013

References

Amaresekere, M. & Henderson, D. (2012). 'Post-Conflict Mental Health in South Sudna: Overview of Common Psychiatric Disorders. Part 1: Depression and Post-traumatic Stress Disorder.' In *South Sudan Medical Journal*, Vol. 1, No. 5, pp. 1–12.

Clancy, M.A. & Hamber, B. (2008). 'Trauma, Peacebuilding, and Development: An Overview of Key Positions and Critical Questions'. Paper presented at the Trauma, Development and Peacebuilding Conference, New Delhi, India, September 9–11. Retrieved 18 August 2015 from: http://www.swisspeace.ch/fileadmin/user_upload/Media/Topics/Dealing_with_the_Past/Resources/Clancy_Mary_Trauma_Peacebuilding_and_Development.pdf.

Common Bond Institute (2014). 'The Catastrophic Trauma Recovery Project'. Retrieved 19 March 2015 from: http://cbiworld.org/ctr/.

Dress, T.P. (2005). *Designing a Peacebuilding Infrastructure: Taking a Systems Approach to the Prevention of Deadly Conflict.* Geneva: The United Nations Non-Governmental Liaison Service.

Eiling, E., Van Diggele-Holtland, M., Van Yperen, T. & Boer, F. (2014). 'Psychosocial Support for Children in the Republic of South Sudan: An Evaluation Outcome'. In *Intervention*, Vol. 12, No. 1, pp. 61–75.

Fuertes, A.B. (2004). 'In Their Own Words: Contextualizing the Discourse of (War) Trauma and Healing'. In *Conflict Resolution Quarterly*, Vol. 21, No. 4, pp. 491–501.

Gallagher, E., Hamber, B. & Joy, E. (2012). 'Perspectives and Possibilities: Mental Health in Post-Agreement Northern Ireland'. In *Shared Space: A Research Journal on Peace, Conflict and Community Relations in Northern Ireland,* Vol. 13, pp. 63–78.

Gasana, S.N. (2008). 'Confronting Conflict and Poverty Through Trauma Healing: Integrating Peace-Building and Development Processes in Rwanda'. In Clark, P. & Kaufman, Z. D. (Eds.)

After Genocide: Transitional Justice, Post-Conflict Reconstruction and Reconciliation in Rwanda and Beyond. London: Hurst & Company, pp. 145–169.
Gawerc, M.I. (2006). 'Peace-building: Theoretical and Concrete Perspectives'. In *Peace and Change*, Vol. 31, pp. 435–478.
Gutlove, P. & Thompson, P. 2006. 'Using Psychosocial Healing in Postconflict Reconstruction'. In Fitzduff, M. & Stout, C.E. (Eds.) *The Psychology of Resolving Global Conflicts: From War to Peace, Volume 3: Interventions* (pp. 185–213). Westport, Con.: Praeger Security International.
Hamber, B., Gallagher, E. & Ventevogel, P. (2014). 'Narrowing the Gap between Psychosocial Practice, Peacebuilding and Wider Social Change: An Introduction to the Special Section in This Issue'. In *Intervention*, Vol. 12, No. 1, pp. 7–15.
Hart, B. (2008). 'Introduction'. In Hart, B. (Ed.) *Peacebuilding in Traumatized Societies.* New York: University Press of America, pp. vii–xi.
Hart, B. & Colo, E. (2014). 'Psychosocial Peacebuilding in Bosnia and Herzegovina: Approaches to Relational and Social Change'. In *Intervention*, Vol. 12, No. 1, pp. 76–87.
Harvey, M. (2007). 'Towards an Ecological Understanding of Resilience'. In *Trauma Survivors: Implications for Theory, Research and Practice.* Harvard Medical School: Victims of Violence Program.
Institute for Justice and Reconciliation (2015). 'Healing Communities, Transforming Society Conference: Exploring the Interconnectedness Between Psycho-Social Needs, Practice and Peacebuilding'. Retrieved 18 August 2015 from: http://ijr.org.za/home/wp-content/uploads/2016/11/IJR-Healing-communities-conference-WEB.pdf.
Inter-Agency Standing Committee (2007). 'IASC Guidelines on Mental Health and Psychosocial Support in Emergency Settings'. Retrieved 18 August 2015 from: http://www.who.int/mental_health/emergencies/guidelines_iasc_mental_health_psychosocial_june_2007.pdf.
Kleinman, A. (1977). 'Depression, Somatization and The "New Cross-Cultural Psychiatry"'. In *Social Science and Medicine*, Vol. 11, pp. 3–10.
Lambourne, W. & Gitau, L. (2013). 'Psychosocial Interventions, Peacebuilding and Development in Rwanda', *Journal of Peacebuilding and Development*. Vol. 8, No. 3, pp. 23–36.
Lambourne, W. & Niyonzima, D. (2015), 'Breaking Cycles of Trauma and Violence: Psychosocial Approaches to Healing and Reconciliation in Burundi'. In Gobodo-Madikizela, P. (Ed.), *Breaking Cycles of Repetition: A Global Dialogue on Historical Trauma and Memory*, Leverkusen: Budrich Academic Press.
LeBaron, M. (2003). *Bridging Cultural Conflicts: A New Approach For a Changing World.* San Francisco: Jossey-Bass.
Lykes, M.B. (2000). 'Possible Contributions of a Psychology of Liberation: Whither Health and Human Rights?' In *Journal of Health Psychology*, Vol. 5, No. 3, pp. 383–397.
Pupavac, V. (2004). 'Psychosocial Interventions and the Demoralization of Humanitarinism'. In *Journal of Biosocial Science*, Vol. 36, No. 4, pp. 491–504.
Ramanathapillai, R. (2006). 'The Politicizing of Trauma: A Case Study of Sri Lanka'. In *Peace and Conflict: Journal of Peace Psychology,* Vol. 12, No. 1, pp. 1–18.
Samuels, K. (2005). 'Post-Conflict Peace-Building and Constitution-Making'. In *Chicago Journal of International Law*, Vol. 6 No. 2, pp. 663–682.
Silove, D. (2004). 'The Challenges facing Mental Health Programs for Post-conflict and Refugee Communities'. In *Prehospital and Disaster Medicine*, Vol. 19, No. 1, pp. 90–96.
Tol, W.A., Barbui, C., Galappatti, A., Silove, D., Betancourt, T.S., Souza, R., Golaz, A. & Van Ommeren, M. (2011). 'Mental Health and Psycho-social Support in Humanitarian Settings: Linking Practice and Research'. In *The Lancet*, Vol. 378, pp. 1581–1591.
Volkan, V. (2001) 'Transgenerational Transmissions and Chosen Traumas: An Aspect of Large-Group Identity'. *Group Analysis.* 34 (1) London: Sage, pp. 79–97. Retrieved 13 July 2015 from: http://gaq.sagepub.com/content/34/1/79.full.pdf+html.
Woodside, D., Santa Barbara, J. & Benner, D. (1999). 'Psychological Trauma and Social Healing in Croatia'. In *Medicine, Conflict and Survival*, Vol. 15, pp. 355–367.

Yoder, C. (2013). 'Trauma-Sensitive Development and Humanitarian Aid'. In *Peacebuilder*. Eastern Mennonite University: Centre for Justice and Peacebuilding, pp. 1–2. Retrieved 13 July 2015 from: http://emu.edu/now/peacebuilder/2013/03/trauma-sensitive-acknowledging-peoples-difficult-experiences-can-help-them-move-forward/.

Zelizer, C. (2008). 'Trauma Sensitive Peace Building: Lessons for Theory and Practice'. In *Africa Peace and Conflict Journal*, Vol. 1, No. 1, pp. 81–94.

Chapter 3
The Lace of Peace's Coat: Understanding Trauma, Peace and Peacebuilding

I sought thee in a secret cave
And ask'd, if Peace were there
A hollow wind did seem to answer, No:
....
This is the lace of Peace's coat:
I will search out the matter.
George Herbert, *Peace*, 1633

3.1 Experiencing Trauma

In June 2014, I participated in a training forum on trauma in which participants were encouraged to contextualize the knowledge to their own situations. A fellow African participant, in an unforgettable outburst expressed to me with frustration, 'What is all this talk about trauma? What is trauma anyway? [There is no term that directly translates to trauma in her African mother tongue or mine.] My grandmother taught me how to move on after facing hard circumstances. These people [the trainers] are going to traumatize us with their talk on trauma! We'd better be careful.' She was serious and visibly angry.

This simple spontaneous expression triggered a deeper reflection on my part about this 'talk on trauma'. How legitimate was it? What did it really mean? What indeed was 'all this talk about trauma'? In my research arising from a concern for the plight of thousands of South Sudanese refugees in Kakuma Refugee Camp, victims of a seemingly unending crisis in their country, and previous research with survivors of the 1994 genocide in Rwanda, I had tended to take the term for granted and run with it, in the same manner that a novice aid worker or missionary lands in a deprived territory and totally believing his/her motives to be completely pure, begins 'helping' the people.

Herman (1997: 33) defines psychological trauma as the sense of being completely overwhelmed by a very stressful event, in which 'the ordinary systems of care that give people a sense of control, connection, and meaning' are destroyed. This sense of overwhelm means that the attachments of family, friendship, love, and

L.W. Gitau, *Trauma-Sensitivity and Peacebuilding*, The Anthropocene: Politik—Economics—Society—Science 12, DOI 10.1007/978-3-319-49803-4_3

community are shattered, and the belief systems that give meaning to human experience are undermined (Herman 1997: 51).

However, beyond Herman's (1997) definition, the meaning of trauma has been analysed, philosophized and politicized to the extent that it has emerged as an indistinct genre requiring deconstruction. This is more so due to the fact that the term, having been conceived, birthed and nurtured in the West, has now come to be applied universally and timelessly to instances where people have experienced events that destroy all sense of security and safety.

This contemplation on the meaning of trauma naturally leads to a philosophical question: Is it the 'talk on trauma' that 'trauma-tizes' an experience (as my colleague remarked), or is trauma an entity existing out there waiting to be experienced by human beings who are so unfortunate as to get to proximity with it and therefore get traumatized by it? In other words, is trauma constructed by human beings or is it a pre-existing phenomenon? This question and its answer has ramifications for the varied experiences of victims and survivors of war atrocities and the consequences of these experiences, as will emerge in the discussion of the experience of the South Sudanese refugees in Kakuma Refugee Camp.

Many philosophers, anthropologists, sociologists and psychologists have pondered this question as they have tried to grapple with the concept of trauma. I will here discuss the deliberations of some of them in an attempt to shed light on the question as it relates to the discussion of the experience of the South Sudanese refugees that follows.

In her universally recognized landmark work *Trauma and Recovery*, Herman (1997) proposes that the understanding of the concept of psychological trauma is provisional, dependent on the political interest of the time, when she says:

> At the moment, the study of psychological trauma seems to be firmly established as a legitimate field of inquiry… But history teaches us that this knowledge could also disappear. Without the context of a political movement, it has never been possible to advance the study of psychological trauma. The fate of this field of knowledge depends upon the fate of the same political movement that inspired and sustained it over the last century (Herman 1997: 32).

If this were the case, then it would mean that without the right political will, the meaning and significance of the concept of trauma would wane and could only be saved by a repeat of what brought it to the fore in the first place, the victims of tragedies 'marching in from the peripheries of the story to demand inclusion' as cited in the forward to Herman (1997: v).

According to the Oxford English Dictionary (1989), the term 'trauma' originates from the Greek word literally meaning 'wound or external bodily injury in general'. As Sharpe (2007) points out, the term was used by Freud in psychoanalysis to describe the events that his free association patients associated with their ailment. Freud seemed to suggest that these events 'are as fractious in the fabric of individuals' self-understandings as the puncturing of skin or breaking of bones in physical traumas' (Sharpe 2007: 2). Deutscher (2007: 10) further summarizes the psychoanalytic sense of the word trauma as 'a condition that derives from the distress and disturbance caused by some sort of wound, physical or emotional, and then becomes repressed rather than lived through and lived out'. The idea of trauma as a wound, in the physical sense, is translated to the understanding of trauma as psychological hurt.

Herman (1997) traces the 'forgotten' history of the study of psychological trauma, which has developed in distinct stages and at each stage, been determined by a particular political movement. The first stage studied hysteria, a psychological disorder associated with women, in the late nineteenth century (Herman 1997: 9–20). This was during the age of the enlightenment, when men sought to prove that secular enlightenment was scientifically and morally superior to religiosity and its associated superstitions. A solution to hysteria was seen to be a demonstration of this superiority.

The second stage was the study of shell shock or combat neurosis, as the psychological disorders that soldiers developed as a result of being involved in war were known (Herman 1997: 20–28). This stage began after the First World War (1914–1918) and grew with force after the Vietnam War (1955–1975). As people became increasingly disillusioned with the negative consequences of war, the psychological trauma associated with war, especially as observed among war veterans, came into public consciousness. Psychiatrists undertook systematic investigations of the psychological effects of war. This development flourished under the antiwar political movement. This eventually led to the acceptance of psychological trauma as a proper, recognisable, medical condition (Herman 1997: 28).

The third stage is the study of sexual and domestic violence. Women's sexual experiences, which had been concealed in the private domain, began being revealed in the public domain, and people became increasingly conscious of the similarities between the psychological effects experienced by survivors of war and those of women who had been sexually abused (Herman 1997: 28–32). This third stage was made possible by the feminist movement that began in the 1970s, which enabled research, documentation, expression and action in relation to sexual assault of women.

The current stage in the development of the study of psychological trauma is largely influenced by the anti-terrorism movement, post September 2001 (9/11) attack on the United States. In the wake of actual and feared terrorist attacks in the twenty-first century, and the reality of ongoing conflicts and wars, especially intra-state, across the world, the term 'trauma' has gained a wide currency (Sharpe 2007). The concept of trauma after mass violence has for instance grown in large bounds in the journalism field. The efforts began by the DART Centre for Journalism and Trauma, a program that started in 1991 with the aim of improving the quality of coverage of traumatic events, and raising awareness of the impact such coverage has on journalists telling the stories, were greatly revamped post 9/11 (Saul 2014). Previously, it had often been thought that journalists needed to be detached and totally objective in order to tell their stories professionally and accurately. Amongst the lessons relearnt and reemphasized post 9/11 were that journalists could be emotional and subjective in conveying their stories, and that indeed the awareness of their own feelings and reactions to the event could help them report the stories more empathetically.

From 1980 when psychological trauma was included in the Diagnostic and Statistical Manual of Mental Disorders (DSM-III) by the American Psychiatric Association (APA) following official recognition of the symptoms as a 'real' diagnosis (Herman 1997: 28), reference to psychological trauma has become almost synonymous with Post Traumatic Stress Disorder (PTSD). The question of how relevant this diagnosis is in different contexts continues to be debated.

The anthropologist, Young (1997: 5), like Herman (1997), discusses the provisional nature of the concept of trauma. He disputes the timelessness and intrinsic quality of trauma, and suggests that 'it is glued together by the practices, technologies and narratives with which it is diagnosed, studied, treated, and represented by various interests, institutions, and moral arguments that mobilized these efforts and resources.' His argument is that trauma is constructed by human beings to fit a particular form and fulfill a specific agenda.

Following Young's (1997) train of thought, Edkins (2003: 43) argues that post-traumatic stress is both historically and geographically specific. She explains this to mean that '…traumatic stress as a possible diagnosis, as something people can be seen and see themselves as suffering from, has become current in a particular time period', and in a particular place, the West. This obviously calls into question the legitimacy of the application of the diagnosis to non-Western societies. This point notwithstanding, the DSM continues to evolve.

The American Psychiatric Association recently (May, 2013) published the fifth edition of the Diagnostic and Statistical Manual of Mental Disorders (DSM-V) which is used by clinicians worldwide as a guide in understanding and treating mental disorders, including PTSD. In this new edition, PTSD is no longer categorized as an anxiety disorder, but is placed in a new category called 'Trauma and Stress-related Disorders', which could help to de-stigmatize it because with this change, PTSD ceases to be seen as an anxiety-related mental illness but rather as a disorder arising from an external event. The diagnostic criteria for PTSD include exposure to a traumatic event such as death, serious injury or sexual violence, intrusion or re-experiencing the event in memories, nightmares or flashbacks, avoidant symptoms such as avoiding any memory of the event, negative alterations in mood or cognitions (which is a new criterion), and increased arousal symptoms which include difficulty in concentrating, irritability, hypervigilance, and being easily startled. The new criteria also include dissociation as a subtype of PTSD, which specifically points to two symptoms: depersonalization or feeling disconnected from oneself, and derealization which is a sense that one's surroundings are not real.

In 2006, a team of 60 African psychiatrists and psychologists attempted to contexualize the American Psychiatric Association's DSM-IV-TR criteria for mental disorders (Ndetei et al. 2006) in *The African Textbook of Clinical Psychiatry and Mental Health*, which has gone a long way in helping to equip mental health workers in Africa with the much needed knowledge and skills to meet the increasing demands for psychological help in African populations. This textbook though, seems to endorse the DSM-IV-TR criteria for PTSD almost to the letter (Ndetei et al. 2006: 222–223), taking it for granted that it is as applicable in African situations as it is in North America or any other place in the world for that matter. The argument is, as a medical condition, of necessity and for credibility, the PTSD diagnosis should fit all people indiscriminately, in much the same way as do diagnoses for physical illnesses such as malaria or diabetes.

This medicalization of trauma could be problematic as it were. While all people belong to the same human species, their experiences and perceptions are mediated by their culture and life circumstances. Bracken (2003), in his presentation of the relationships between trauma, meaning and culture, argues that this medical framing

> …can cover up as well as illuminate the reasons for our pain and suffering. It is often presented to patients as 'the truth' of their condition and serves to silence other possibilities. Psychiatric diagnosis is often little more than a simplification of a complex reality and by formulating an individual's experience in terms of pathology it can be profoundly disempowering and stigmatizing (Bracken 2003: 4).

Bracken argues that a person's experience of his or her illness is not secondary to the medical diagnosis, but has a validity of its own.

The question of meaning is crucial, for it appears that it is in the 'gluing together' of the concept of trauma (Young 1997), the 'advancing' of the study of psychological trauma (Herman 1997), the 'framing' of what trauma is (Bracken 2003), and the manner of the 'talk on trauma' as pointed out by my African colleague, that the issue really lies. The work of the German philosopher Martin Heidegger and his approach to the question of meaning, and Bracken's (2003) discourse, shed light on the issue with the meaning of trauma.

Heidegger's (1927/1996: 2–3) standpoint underscores the idea that knowledge is dependent on experiential evidence. We cannot dissect existence, how we experience the world, and separate it into distinct parts identifiable as entities in their own right. The essence of 'Being' is as a whole. In the same vein, Bracken (2003: 87–89) argues that our practical involvement in life is primary, in fact essential, to 'being' human, and being human, we give meaning to the world we inhabit. The meaning we give to the world is based on the social world we live in.

The world we experience then is not neutral. We encounter the world in this state of embeddedness, which makes it meaningful to us (Heidegger 1927/1996; Bracken 2003). Our thoughts, words and feelings are part of this world that we encounter, and are culturally embedded. The social and cultural setting in relation to trauma is thus important, since the way an individual or a community's world is meaningful to them will determine how they react to an event. This offers a foundation for the understanding of the culturally embedded ways in which the South Sudanese refugees in Kakuma Refugee Camp understand their experiences, as discussed in this book. These culturally-embedded ways include the collective nature of the experience of trauma, as discussed in the next section.

3.1.1 Collective Trauma

The concept of collective trauma refers to the 'shared injuries to a population's social, cultural, and physical ecologies' (Saul 2014: 1). The impact of a traumatic event, such as mass violence, is experienced in relationships in families, communities and societies at large. The social and cultural systems are rendered dysfunctional, and patterns of dependency, paternalism, powerlessness, and social fragmentation ensue (Kantowitz/Riak 2008). While trauma is primarily individually experienced, the experience is in turn 'socially and culturally mediated and determined' (Culbertson/Pouligny 2007: 271). It is not just the individual, but culture itself that is the casualty of the mass violence.

Sarat et al. (2007: 7) trace the origin of the conceptualization of trauma as a collective phenomenon to the second half of the twentieth century, with the emergence of the critique on liberalism and its overemphasis on individualism. The liberal worldview was especially critiqued for being unable to deal with the horrors of the Holocaust, and this led to an examination of the collective nature of the ideologies on which racism and prejudice were established, as well as the collective nature of the resultant traumas. Sarat et al. (2007: 7) point out that as a result:

> Emphasis on social construction and the use of cultural narratives as a means to explain the self, produced a shift in trauma analysis by tying it to broad social structures (including structural violence) and moving it away from the individual as a primary unit of inquiry. Instead, collective identity becomes the unit of analysis and a group that shares an identity such as ethnicity, nationality, gender, or religion is considered as the primary unit that experiences trauma.

The issue of identity is closely tied to the experience of trauma. Identity is among the first casualties of traumatic events. As such, after a traumatic event, the survivors are firmly engaged in attempting to restore their identity. Volkan (2001: 79) introduces the concept of 'chosen trauma' as one component of this identity. By chosen trauma, Volkan means 'the shared representation of a massive trauma that the group's ancestors suffered at the hand of an enemy'. During this past event, the group may have suffered loss and experienced shame, humiliation and helplessness, and was unable 'to mourn its losses of people, land or prestige' (Volkan 2001: 87).

This chosen trauma is reawakened or reactivated when a group regresses socially, due to loss of basic trust. Saul (2014: 4) similarly alludes to this reawakening arguing that traumatic events easily lead to the opening up of 'previously existing fault lines of racism and other forms of discrimination, social and economic inequalities, and prior historical traumas'. Volkan (2001: 79) gives an example of postcolonial Africa among others, where, after the colonial powers retreated, groups were engaged in exaggerated attempts at defining and redefining themselves as a people, often involving violent conflict between tribes that had a lot in common but continued to insist that they were inherently different. This may for instance be seen in the manner of the civil wars in South Sudan discussed in Chap. 1. It is in this effort to protect their identity that the collective nature of the trauma experienced is evident. The chosen trauma becomes woven into the social fabric of the whole group, as it defines what they experience collectively.

The concept of collective trauma becomes particularly relevant in re-imagining peace after violent conflict. The group's ability to engage in peacebuilding activities is impacted negatively and needs to be restored. In the same way that a group has suffered trauma collectively and social systems have been disrupted, subsequent social structures and cultural categories can be collectively reconstructed (Culbertson/Pouligny 2007: 281). This calls for the need to view interventions for survivors of violent conflict with a double lens, the culturally respectful lens (Keane 2003: 358; Baron et al. 2003: 250), and the trauma lens (Hart 2014). Keane (2003: 358) underscores the need to collaborate with communities and co-opt the leadership of communities in developing interventions that are culturally sensitive and effective. Maynard (1997: 211) proposes the use of 'communalization', which she defines as 'the act of sharing traumatic experiences, perceptions, resulting emotions, and responses with other people in a safe environment' as an important part of the healing from trauma.

Collectively, the capacities of the group to engage in productive activities can be restored through engaging the members of the community in participatory community development processes, which, as Kantowitz/Riak (2008: 8) suggest, helps to give the communities and groups agency and thus contribute to the healing of trauma.

Saul (2014) similarly underscores the need to recognize and strengthen the community's resilience after collective trauma and argues:

> As collective trauma refers to disruptions of relationships at all levels of human systems, recovery then involves collective processes of readjustment and adaptation and the mobilization of capacities for resilience in families and communities (Saul 2014: 6).

Understanding trauma as a collective phenomenon thus leads to a conceptualization of the healing of trauma, the meaning of peace, and subsequent peacebuilding activities as a collective issue, involving relationships, as discussed in the sections that follow.

3.2 Defining Peace

Peace is elusive, seemingly unattainable. Yet for centuries, human beings have been seeking to understand it, to know it, grasp it, experience it, and spread it. In an attempt at grasping the meaning of peace, Webel (2012) ascribes both earthly and other-worldly features to peace. He describes it as 'both a means of personal and collective ethical transformation and an aspiration to cleanse the planet of human-inflicted destruction' (Webel 2012: 69). Despite the attempt by psychologists and philosophers to illuminate the subject of peace for over a century, a deep understanding of peace remains inchoate. Like light, it is intangible, but all the more apparent and easier to define in its absence (Webel 2012: 72).

The complexity and indistinctness of the concept of peace, however, does not discourage us from trying to understand it. For as Richmond (2007: 204) observes, 'Where people's lives are at stake there is little more that can be done than try, learn, and try again, aware, but unaware, enlightened but still blind'. And so we continue to grapple on, not knowing, and not having any certainty, but with the belief and hope that even the little we know and continue to discover will in some way contribute to alleviating the situation of those affected by violent conflict.

'The peace that I can see is you', said Amuka,[1] one of the participants of this research, when I asked her what she understood by the term peace. Amuka had left her home in South Sudan fourteen years previously, after her parents and her husband had been killed in the civil war. She had sought refuge in Kakuma refugee camp in Kenya, where she had remarried, and after the birth of two children, her second husband had also died. Now she was lonely and wanted someone to visit and talk with her. In a small, personal way, I was 'her peace'.

On December 10 1948, Eleanor Roosevelt said of Human Rights in her speech during the adoption of a resolution endorsing the Universal Declaration of Human Rights before the General Assembly of the United Nations:

> Where, after all, do universal human rights begin? In *small places, close to home - so close and so small that they cannot be seen on any maps of the world* (italics added) … Such are the places where every man, woman, and child seeks equal justice, equal opportunity, equal dignity without discrimination. Unless these rights have meaning there, they have little meaning anywhere. Without concerted citizen action to uphold them close to home, we shall look in vain for progress in the larger world (Roosevelt 1948).

The same can be said about peace as of human rights. Peace begins in small places close to home, and unless peace has meaning in these small places, it may not have meaning anywhere else. For Amuka, peace began right there, where she was, sitting on a mat outside her hut in hot, dry and dusty Kakuma, and me sitting next to her, listening to her story.

Peace can be defined as both a process and a goal: a process in the sense of an aspiration towards an optimum, idealistic point, and a goal in the sense of an achievable global objective (Richmond 2012: 36–38). The ontological shakiness of the term peace seems to match the deficiency of the experience of peace. It is perhaps this murkiness of meaning that causes peace to appear to have been on trial throughout history as Cortright (2012: 118) observes, 'standing like a forlorn defendant before the court of established opinion, misunderstood and maligned on all sides'. If peace cannot stand up for itself, why should others stand for it, this critique seems to argue.

And so peace has tried to 'stand up for itself' as it were, by seeking to establish itself as a legitimate discipline in its own right. Peace studies began being identified as a separate field of inquiry during the first decades after World War II. In the mid-1970s, Johan Galtung advanced the concepts of positive peace and negative peace. Negative peace, according to Galtung, refers to the absence of direct

[1]Interview with Amuka on 3 July 2013. See Appendix 3.1.

violence and the absence of massive killings of humans. Positive peace, by contrast, involves the absence of structural violence which includes suffering caused by economic and political structures of exploitation and repression, and the absence of the cultural violence that legitimizes direct and structural violence (Galtung 1975, 1976).

A reflection of peace as a multilayered phenomenon may illuminate the understanding of peace further, and render it more accessible. With this understanding, peace is conceived as having different levels that form a whole: The inner peace core, the middle interpersonal and intercommunal peace layer, and the outer national and international peace layer. The layers form a complex web towards achieving peace. The web comprises in the different approaches generally used to conceptualize peace. Richmond (2007: 185) identifies the internal and external binary of peace, which demonstrates the disparity between local and international actors' understanding of peace. This is closely related to the top-down and bottom-up construction of peace. Peace as a top-down construction means its achievement depends on international or state-level official actors, while peace as a bottom-up construction, means it is derived from individuals, communities and civil society actors (Richmond 2007: 188).

The interplay of the different layers of peace is further illustrated by a description of how the inner personal core and the intercommunal layer affect the national and international layers. The Institute of Economics and Peace (2012) notes that a higher per capita income and high levels of well-being and economic sustainability are a mark of a peaceful society. Yet, as Gasana (2008: 156) notes, when people are struggling with inner pain as a result of the atrocities of war, they become dysfunctional and unproductive. Drawing on his own personal experience as a survivor of the 1994 genocide in Rwanda and a peace and development practitioner, Gasana (2008: 145) argues that there is need for emotional healing from the trauma caused by war in order to 'recover functional capacities and the creativity necessary for social and economic productivity'.

From this cyclical state of affairs then, while the nation demands of its citizens to be economically productive so that it can be said to be at peace in the global arena, the citizens 'demand' healing from what they have suffered in order to be at peace and therefore economically productive. Who will go first then? Asking survivors of conflict and mass violence how they feel and what they perceive to be barriers to peace may help us understand this seemingly paradoxical relationship.

With the understanding of peace as a multilayered concept, it seems expedient to pay careful attention to the initial layers, in order to lay a firm foundation for the eventual layers. The attention to detail given to the intricate and elaborate designs of the foundations of the Burj Khalifa in Dubai, the world's tallest building (Emporis Research 2014), give a good illustration of what is needed to build sustainable peace, seemingly the world's 'tallest' aspiration. For the foundation of the Burj Khalifa, a thorough assessment was carried out to ensure that piled foundations would be appropriate to hold the construction. A number of analyses were used to assess the response of the foundation, and an overall stability assessment was done.

The preparations, time, costs, concentration and commitment that went into the establishment of these foundations are significantly elaborate (Poulos/Bunce 2008).

A similar level of concentration and commitment is needed for the establishment of the foundations of peace, at the individual and communal levels. During and after violent conflict, the survivors, as individuals and communities, need to rebuild their lives from the inside out. Concentrating on brokering peace for the nation by international bodies without handling the emotional and psychological effects of the atrocities on the individuals and communities affected appears like building the towers and spires of the Burj Khalifa without laying the foundations in the detail described.

Understanding peace as relationship, contributes to the idea of building the foundations that are necessary in helping individuals and communities negotiate the negative effects of mass violence and to be well on the path to peace. The Jewish philosopher Martin Buber's notion of 'I and Thou' (Buber 1922/2002) offers a basis for understanding peace as relationship. Buber posits that there cannot be an 'I' without a 'You', and the 'I' can only be fully a person, and exist in entirety, in relation to the 'You'. In a sense, the 'I' and the 'You' are one, and life and experience loses meaning if this oneness is dismantled as happens in situations of violent conflict.

Similarly, Lederach argues that relationship is 'both the basis of the conflict and its long-term solution', and reconciliation of necessity needs to involve 'mechanisms that engage the sides of a conflict with each other as humans-in-relationship' (Lederach 1997: 26).

Relationship is thus central to the definition of peace as discussed in this book.

3.3 Understanding Peacebuilding

Peacebuilding, a term that came into existence through the work of Johan Galtung, 'Three Approaches to Peace: Peacekeeping, Peacemaking and Peacebuilding' (1976) refers to the mechanisms and activities put in place in order to address the 'root causes' of violent conflict, and explore ways of managing and resolving conflict. This is in an attempt to transform a society from a state of violence to peace. The term however came into the international realm through the former United Nations Secretary-General Boutros Boutros-Ghali in *An Agenda for Peace* published in 1992, when he defined it as 'action to identify and support structures which will tend to strengthen and solidify peace in order to avoid relapse into conflict' (Boutros-Ghali 1992).

This definition and scope of peacebuilding was expanded in the *Supplement to An Agenda for Peace* published in 1995, to encompass all phases of conflict, and again in the *2000 Report of the Panel on United Nations Peace Operations* (the Brahimi Report) as

> activities undertaken on the far side of conflict to reassemble the foundations of peace and provide the tools for building on those foundations something that is more than just the absence of war (Global Policy Forum 2000).

In 2007, the UN Secretary General's Policy Committee agreed on the following conceptual basis for peacebuilding:

> Peacebuilding involves a range of measures targeted to reduce the risk of lapsing or relapsing into conflict by strengthening national capacities at all levels for conflict management, and to lay the foundations for sustainable peace and development. Peacebuilding strategies must be coherent and tailored to specific needs of the country concerned, based on national ownership, and should comprise a carefully prioritized, sequenced, and therefore relatively narrow set of activities aimed at achieving the above objectives (UN 2010).

Despite all these developments, peacebuilding remains 'a fragile undertaking with mixed results' (Tschirgi 2004: i). The focus of international peacebuilding is chiefly on the relationship with the government of the affected country, not on the local actors and structures (Da Costa/Karlsrud 2012; Paris 2004). This kind of peacebuilding has been criticized for having a state-centric bias as opposed to having a 'people-centred, locally owned' approach (Baker/Scheye 2007: 503). The central task is seen as building the state itself, which depends upon a common societal consensus on the values and laws underpinning the state, as much as on basic, functioning institutions. As Baker/Scheye (2007) further note, this focus seems to be ignoring the fact that state-building endeavours may be illegitimate in the eyes of the majority of the population, and that the separation and displacement caused by war and other mass violence may make it impossible to identify a 'common societal consensus'.

South Sudan, as with many other societies emerging from conflict, may benefit from fostering a 'civil peace' which requires individual agency and a focus on what Richmond (2007: 215) has called 'emancipatory' peacebuilding. As Richmond (2007: 102) argues, the original social justice goals of the liberal model emphasized in peace studies theory have been undermined in the 'contemporary peacebuilding project' in which multidimensional peacekeeping has given way to state-building, and the welfare and well-being of the populations affected by the conflict have become marginalized. Goetschel/Hagmann (2009: 57) pointedly refer to the remoteness of such peacebuilding projects to the local communities, the so-called beneficiaries, who are rarely involved in the definition of what peace is or should be.

The international approach to peacebuilding, reflected in various UN definitions, is based on the concept of 'liberal peace' which views political and economic liberalization as the remedies of violent conflict, and posits promotion of human rights, democracy, elections, constitutionalism, rule of law, property rights, good governance, and neo-liberal economics as part of the peacebuilding strategy (Tschirgi 2004: 5). According to Richmond (2007: 183), this liberal peace has been deemed universal and attainable

> … if the correct methods are concertedly and consistently applied by a plethora of different actors working on the basis of an agreed peacebuilding consensus, and focusing on the regimes, structures, and institutions required at multiple levels of analysis and in multiple issue areas by liberal governance.

This approach seems to raise debates about hegemony, with clearly defined roles of interveners (the international actors) as the superior actors, and the recipients of the intervention as the inferior actors.

The challenge of what approaches work at different levels and contexts of peacebuilding remains. It seems prudent to appreciate the complexity of the field of peacebuilding and not to generalize or be quick to dismiss varying attempts at building peace after violent conflict as completely ineffective. Paris (2011), while critiquing the critiques of liberal peacebuilding, warns against an oversimplification of the moral complexitys of international peacebuilding, and calls for a more thorough evaluation of its various benefits. He argues:

> It is a truism to observe that there are elements of 'folly' in every human institution, including international peacebuilding. If we accept this as a given, the more important ethical issue is whether international peacebuilding, viewed as a whole, not just in fragments, remains a justified and worthwhile enterprise. Among other considerations, answering this question requires careful assessment of possible alternative courses of action (or inaction). To arrive at sweeping moral judgments about peacebuilding based on fragmentary analysis is not only methodologically suspect, but it is ethically problematic in itself, given how much is at stake in debates over how and when to provide assistance to societies emerging from conflict (Paris 2011: 46).

It is with this sensitivity to the complexities of the whole spectrum of approaches to peacebuilding that we take a cautious outlook at the peacebuilding process and do not lay claim to the answer to the problem of peacebuilding, but rather seek to underscore an important addition to the approaches to make the realization of peace after mass violence more feasible.

The field of peacebuilding is still in the process of identifying the various pieces of the puzzle that are needed for building sustainable peace, and how each piece contributes to the process and is part of an integrated whole (Jeong 2005: 14). Trauma-sensitivity in interventions for survivors of violent conflict is one such piece. The work of the peacebuilding practitioner and scholar, John Paul Lederach sheds further light to understanding the process of peacebuilding, in its different components.

3.3.1 Peacebuilding Imagined

Lederach's (1997: 20) defines peacebuilding as 'a comprehensive concept that encompasses, generates, and sustains the full array of processes, approaches, and stages needed to transform conflict toward more sustainable, peaceful relationships' most aptly captures the focus of this book. Lederach conceptualizes peace as a social construct, which requires the process of building. The building process of necessity involves careful consideration of the materials needed, investing in getting the materials ready for the construction, careful deliberation of the architectural design to be applied, laying the foundation, attention to detail in the finish work, and continued maintenance (Lederach 1997), much in the same way as detailed in the description of the building of the Burj Khalifa (Poulos/Bunce 2008).

The philosophy of peacebuilding adopted in this book is derived from Lederach's (2005) subsequent work, *The Moral Imagination: The Art and Soul of Peacebuilding.* While acknowledging that peacebuilding is indeed a complex task, Lederach (2005) seeks to embrace simplicity in identifying four simple disciplines that form 'the moral imagination' and when practiced make peacebuilding possible. These four disciplines are relationship, paradoxical curiosity, creativity, and risk (Lederach 2005: 34).

On relationships, Lederach observes that even in the midst of violent conflict, it is possible to imagine the ties that bind people together as human beings, thus transcending and breaking the barriers that separate them as enemies. The second part of Talia's dream in Chap. 1 illustrates this realization, when she came to see the vulnerability of her pursuer, identified with him, and gave him her shoes.

This interconnectedness of people with their enemies, Lederach calls a 'web of relationship' (Lederach 2005: 34–35), and the essence of peacebuilding involves 'the art of web making and web watching'. In other words, peacebuilding efforts need to concentrate on understanding the dynamics and potentials of this web, and tapping into them. Relationships provide the context for the realization, the 'moral imagination' that '... ultimately the quality of our life is dependent on the quality of life of others... that the well-being of our grand-children is directly tied to the well-being of our enemy's grandchildren' (Lederach 2005: 35). This interconnectedness is also reflected in the African social ethic of Ubuntu, which means 'one is a person through others', a unifying notion, according to which all persons are interconnected (Gade 2013).

Relationships are central to humanity. Building peace is an effort to restore relationships that violent conflict has endeavoured to destroy: an effort to restore humanity. In his exploration of what makes us human and driven to care about other human beings subjected to violent conflict and other atrocities, Rorty (1999) concludes that it is neither rationality as advanced by Plato, nor a moral obligation of all human beings as posited by Kant, but rather the capacities for friendship, relationships, and sentimentality. He argues these capacities help us 'to tolerate, and even to cherish ... people whose appearance or habits or beliefs at first seemed an insult to our own moral identity, our sense of the limits of permissible human variation' (Rorty 1999: 80). In a simple way, Talia demonstrates this in her attitude toward her 'enemy' at the end.

The second discipline, paradoxical curiosity, Lederach (2005: 36) defines as the ability to 'rise above dualistic polarities'. This involves an appreciation and respect for the complexity of issues in the conflict context, an aversion to putting things in either/or categories or containers and an inquisitiveness that allows for multiple and even contradictory social realities. Again, like with the web of relationships, this discipline calls for effort in mobilizing this imagination. This paradoxical curiosity is for instance reflected in situations where perpetrators in a conflict end up becoming victims and seeking refuge alongside the people they fought. Sometimes those who had been on opposite sides of the conflict have to live as neighbours in a refugee camp, and share amenities. Paradoxical curiosity involves avoiding quick conclusions, suspending judgement, embracing ambiguity and exploring the contradictions presented for the possibility of a value that supersedes the contradictions (Lederach 2005: 36–37).

The third discipline is the creative act. According to Lederach, this is the discipline through which the moral imagination is expressed. Since it is still an imagination, the notion can only be expressed by going beyond what is experienced, while speaking to it at the same time, as is the nature of poetry, fine art, music and creative writing. A story is told of a poet who would publicly condemn the injustices of his intolerant government again and again in his public poetry recitals. Each time, the police officers would come to arrest him for disloyalty two or three months after the incident of his recital. Apparently it took his government that long to figure out what he was exactly saying against the government! Lederach (2005: 38) defines artists as

> … people who live on the thresholds of the communities they inhabit, from whence the pulse of their lifework emerges and to which they speak. However, by being on the edge they also pose a threat for they push the edges of what is thought to be real and possible.

This discipline requires providing space for the creative act, and believing that it is possible even in settings of violence. This act provides a turning point, creating 'the vision and belief that the future is not the slave of the past and the birth of something new is possible' (Lederach 2005: 39).

The 2012 documentary film *Sweet Dreams* about the Rwandan women's drumming troupe *Ingoma Nshya* exemplifies the creative act as envisioned by Lederach (2005: 38), 'pushing the edges of what is thought to be real and possible'. The unusual women's drumming troupe was founded by playwright Odile Katese with women from both sides of the 1994 genocide (though women in Rwanda were traditionally not allowed to drum), and led to the opening of an ice-cream store in 2010, which also brings together people from both sides of the genocide. Foudras (2013) wrote about it in his review:

> Although the 1994 genocide and its aftermath have been explored extensively in both narrative and nonfiction films over the past decade, *Sweet Dreams* nevertheless forges its own path dwelling less on the violent crimes of the past than on the *small but meaningful ways* [italics added] in which a once-divided people are working to rebuild the social and psychological health of their country (Foudras 2013).

It is these 'small but meaningful ways' that may help in building peace in a society ravaged by conflict. These ways are of necessity derived from an involved understanding of the experiences and perceptions of the people involved in the conflict.

The fourth and final discipline is the willingness to take a risk. This involves stepping into the unknown without having an assurance that things will turn right, but doing it all the same. In the context of violent conflict, the reality, what is known is the conflict, and the unknown, the mystery is peace. Only an 'imagination' or vision of what can be, what is possible, can help people to engage in activities that may lead to peace. An emphasis on trauma-sensitivity in the interventions received by survivors of violent conflict, involves taking a risk as it entails people opening up their hearts and risking being hurt. By agreeing to be interviewed, the survivors take a risk, exposing their pain and hurt as they express what they went through during the conflict.

3.4 Conclusion

The study of psychological trauma developed in distinct stages, and each stage was determined by a particular political movement. A discussion of the work of the German philosopher Martin Heidegger and Bracken's (2003) discourse on Heidegger's work, in relation to the question of 'Being', sheds further light on the meaning and experience of trauma, and the concept of collective trauma demonstrates the culturally-embedded ways in which trauma is understood.

Peace is understood as both a process and a goal. The indistinctness of a peace definition is seen to be related to the deficiency of the experience of peace. The development of peace studies has been an attempt at solidifying the concept of peace as a discipline. Peace as understood by many different actors is further seen as multilayered and intersubjective. Finally, peace is seen as relationship, as postulated by the Jewish philosopher Martin Buber in his 'I-Thou' philosophy, and the peace scholar Lederach.

An understanding of the term peacebuilding remains fragile, and this poses challenges to understanding what approaches work at different levels and in different contexts. There is need for an appreciation of the complexity of the field, in attempting to examine the pieces of the puzzle needed to build peace. Lederach's (2005) concept of 'the moral imagination' captures the essense of peacebuilding, identified in the four simple disciplines relationship, paradoxical curiosity, creativity, and risk (Lederach 2005: 34).

Appendix 3.1

Pseudonym	M/F	Ethnic group	Age	Duration of stay in the camp	Brief details	Date of interview
Amuka	F	Dinka	35	14 years	Walked to Kakuma, escaping both the war in South Sudan and an abusive husband. Married again in the camp and husband died. Lives with her two children in the camp	3rd July 2013

References

Baker, B. & Scheye, E. (2007). 'Multi-layered Justice and Security Delivery in Post-Conflict and Fragile States'. In *Conflict, Security and Development* Vol. 7, No. 4, pp. 503–528.

Baron, N., Jensen, S.B. & de Jong, T.V.M. (2003). 'Refugees and Internally Displaced People'. In Green, B.L., Friedman, M.J., de Jong, T.V.M., et al. (Eds.) *Trauma Interventions in War and Peace.* New York: Kluwer Academic/Plenum Publishers, pp. 243–270.

Boutros-Ghali, B. (1992). 'An Agenda For Peace'. Retrieved January 25 2015 from: http://www.unrol.org/files/a_47_277.pdf.

Bracken, P. (2003). *Trauma: Culture, Meaning and Philosophy.* London: Whurr Publishers.

Buber, M. (1922) *The Martin Buber Reader: Essential Writings.* In Biemann, A.D. (Ed.) (2002). New York: Palgrave Macmillan.

Cortright, D. (2012). 'What is Peace?' In Webel, C.P. & Johansen, J. (Eds.) *Peace and Conflict Studies: A Reader.* London: Routledge, pp. 118–131.

Culbertson, R. & Pouligny, B. (2007). 'Re-imagining peace after mass crime: A dialogical exchange between insider and outsider knowledge'. In Pouligny, B., Chesterman, S. & Schnabel, A. (Eds.) *After Mass Crime: Rebuilding States and Communities.* Tokyo: United Nations University Press, pp. 271–287.

Da Costa, D.F. & Karlsrud, J. (2012). 'Contextualising Liberal Peacebuilding for Local Circumstances: UNMISS and Local Peacebuilding In South Sudan'. In *Journal of Peacebuilding and Development,* Vol. 7, No. 2, pp. 53–66.

Deutscher, M. (2007). 'Thinking Trauma'. In Sharpe, M., Noonan, M. & Freddi, J. (Eds.) *Trauma, History, Philosophy.* Newcastle, UK: Cambridge Scholars Publishing, pp. 10–22.

Edkins, J. (2003). *Trauma and the Memory of Politics.* Cambridge: Cambridge University Press.

Emporis Research (2014). 'The World's Tallest Buildings'. Retrieved 9 April 2015 from: http://www.emporis.com/statistics/worlds-tallest-buildings.

Foudras, S. (2013), 'Film Review' *Sweet Dreams.* Variety. Retrieved January 25 2015 from: http://variety.com/2013/film/reviews/film-review-sweet-dreams-1200800701/.

Gade, C. B.N. (2013) 'Ubuntu and Restorative Justice: Addressing the Strife and Divisions of the Past in Post-Apartheid South Africa'. A PhD Thesis. Aarhus University, Denmark.

Galtung, J. (1975). *Essays in Peace Research,* Volume I. Copenhagen. Christian Ejlers.

Galtung, J. (1976). 'Three Approaches to Peace: Peacekeeping, Peacemaking, and Peacebuilding'. In *Peace, War and Defense: Essays in Peace Research,* Vol. 2. pp. 297–298.

Gasana, S.N. (2008). 'Confronting Conflict and Poverty Through Trauma Healing: Integrating Peace-Building and Development Processes in Rwanda'. In Clark, P. & Kaufman, Z.D. (Eds.)

After Genocide: Transitional Justice, Post-Conflict Reconstruction and Reconciliation in Rwanda and Beyond. London: Hurst & Company, pp. 145–169.
Global Policy Forum (2000). 'Brahimi Report'. Retrieved January 26 2015 from: https://www.globalpolicy.org/security-council/peacekeeping/peacekeeping-reform/40960-the-brahimi-report-and other un documents.html.
Goetschel, L. & Hagmann, T. (2009). 'Civilian Peacebuilding: Peace by Bureaucratic means?' In *Conflict, Security and Development* Vol. 9, No. 1, pp. 55–73.
Hart, B. (2014). PAX 692 Trauma Sensitive Practice and Programming. 'Peacebuilding Wheel: A Model for Social Reconstruction after Complex and Violent Conflict'. Lecture notes. Summer Peacebuilding Institute 2014, Eastern Mennonite University, pp. 1–9.
Heidegger, M. (1996). *Being and Time.* New York: Harper & Row. (Original work published 1927).
Herman, J. (1997). *Trauma and Recovery.* New York: Basic Books.
Institute for Economics and Peace: Global Peace Index (2012). '2011 Methodology, results and findings.' In Webel, C.P. & Johansen, J. (Eds.) *Peace and Conflict Studies: A Reader.* London: Routledge, pp. 46–64.
Lederach, J.P. (1997). *Building Sustainable Peace: Sustainable Reconciliation in Divided Societies.* Washington D.C.: United States Institute of Peace Press.
Lederach, J.P. (2005). *The Moral Imagination: The Art and Soul of Building Peace.* New York: Oxford University Press.
Jeong, H.-W. (2005). *Peacebuilding in Postconflict Societies: Strategy and Process.* London: Lynne Rienner Publishers.
Kantowitz, R. & Riak, A. (2008). 'Critical Links between Peacebuilding and Trauma Healing: A Holistic Framework for Fostering Community Development'. In Hart, B. (Ed.) *Peacebuilding in Traumatized Societies.* Lanham: University Press of America, pp. 3–26.
Keane, T.M. (2003). 'A Call to Action: Responding to Social and Humanitarian Crises'. In Green, B.L, Friedman, M.J., de Jong, J.T.V.M., Solomon, S.D., Keane, T.M., Fairbank, J.A., Donelan, B. & Frey-Wouters, E. (Eds.) *Trauma Interventions in War and Peace: Prevention, Practice and Policy.* New York: Kluwer Academic/Plenum Publishers, pp. 351–362.
Maynard, K.A. (1997). 'Rebuilding Community: Psychosocial Healing, Reintegration, and Reconciliation at the Grassroots Level'. In Kumar, K. (Ed.) *Rebuilding Societies After Civil War: Critical Roles for International Assistance.* London: Lynne Rienner Publishers, pp. 183–203.
Ndetei, D.M, Szabo, C.P, Okasha, T. & Mburu, J. (2006) The African Textbook of Clinical Psychiatry and Mental Health. Nairobi: The African Medical Research Foundation.
Oxford English Dictionary (1989). *Oxford English Dictionary: The definitive record of the English language,* 2nd Ed. Oxford: Oxford University Press. Retrieved 13 July 2015 from: http://www.oed.com.ezproxy1.library.usyd.edu.au/view/Entry/205242?redirectedFrom=trauma#eid.
Paris, R. (2011) 'Critiques of Liberal Peace'. In Campbell, S., Chandler, D. & Sabaratnam, M. (Eds.) *A Liberal Peace?* London: Zed Books, pp. 31–51.
Poulos, H.G. & Bunce, G. (2008). 'Foundations design for the Burj Dubai—the World's Tallest Building'. Retrieved January 16 2015 from: http://www.geomarc.it/Poulos_&_Bunce_2008.pdf.
Richmond, O.P. (2007). *The Transformation of Peace.* New York: Palgrave Macmillan.
Roosevelt, E. (1948). Speech on the Adoption of the Universal Declaration of Human Rights. Retrieved 16 January 2015 from: http://www.americanrhetoric.com/speeches/eleanorrooseveltdeclarationhumanrights.htm.
Rorty, R. (1999). 'Human Rights, Rationality and Sentimentality'. In Savic, O. (Ed.) *The Politics of Human Rights.* London: Verso, pp. 67–83.
Sarat, A., Davidovitch, N., & Alberstein, M. (2007). 'Trauma and Memory: Between Individual and Collective Experiences'. In Sarat, A., Davidovitch, N. & Alberstein, M. (Eds.) *Trauma and Memory: Reading, Healing and Making Law.* Stanford, CA: Stanford University Press, pp. 3–18.
Saul, J. (2014). *Collective Trauma, Collective Healing: Promoting Community Resilience in the Aftermath of Disaster.* New York: Routledge.

Sharpe, M. (2007). 'Introduction: Why Trauma Now?' In Sharpe, M., Noonan, M. & Freddi, J. (Eds.) *Trauma, History, Philosophy.* Newcastle, UK: Cambridge Scholars Publishing, pp. 1–9.

Tschirgi, N. (2004). 'Post-Conflict Peacebuilding Revisited: Achievements, Limitations, Challenges'. New York: International Peacebuilding Academy, Peacebuilding Forum Conference.

United Nations (2010). 'UN Peacebuilding: an Orientation'. Retrieved January 25 2015 from: http://www.un.org/en/peacebuilding/pbso/pdf/peacebuilding_orientation.pdf.

Volkan, V. (2001) 'Transgenerational Transmissions and Chosen Traumas: An Aspect of Large-Group Identity'. *Group Analysis.* 34 (1) London: Sage, pp. 79–97. Retrieved 13 July 2015 from: http://gaq.sagepub.com/content/34/1/79.full.pdf+html.

Webel, C.P. (2012). 'Thinking Peace'. In Webel, C.P. & Johansen, J. (Eds.) *Peace and Conflict Studies: A Reader.* London: Routledge, pp. 65–74.

Young, A. (1997). *Harmony of Illusions: Inventing Posttraumatic Stress Disorder.* Princeton, New Jersey: Princeton University Press.

Chapter 4
Traumatic Experiences of South Sudanese Refugees

The slow, brown, resistless currents of the Congo, the white wrath of Nile cataracts... create and destroy and create anew out of what they destroy...

Phillip Caputo, *Acts of Faith*, 2005, p. 5

4.1 Traumatic Experiences in South Sudan

4.1.1 Torture and Death of Loved Ones: 'They Cut Him to Pieces'

Participants painfully recalled the circumstances that led to their coming to the camp, and loved ones dying. Miriam, a young woman from the Nuba community, expressed in excruciating detail, and with a force of emotion rarely expressed elsewhere in the interviews, the account of her father's murder and the inhumanity of the act. During the interview, Miriam repeated several times how the killers cut up her father's flesh and scattered it about 'like the flesh of a goat':

> *My father was taking the cattle to the river, to take water. And then some people who were riding on camels, and I guess they were the Arabs*[1] *found my father and shot him, and cut his head with a panga into pieces such that his flesh was like the flesh of a goat.... I was still young but I remember what they did to my father... Eeh I saw, I saw all that happen. I just went and found they had made him like goat's meat ... And I was just crying. I could tell the head was my father's but the rest of the body I could not tell that it was my father....*[2]

Another story of inhuman treatment is related by Grace,[3] a 42 year old woman from the Acholi community, who describes how the killers tied a dog to the back of her father, suspecting him of being a traitor, beat the dog and had the dog maul her father to death.

[1]'The Arabs', as used by Miriam and other participants, refer to Northern Sudanese.
[2]Interview with Miriam on 13 July 2013. See Appendix 4.1.
[3]Interview with Grace on 17 July 2013. See Appendix 4.1.

L.W. Gitau, *Trauma-Sensitivity and Peacebuilding*, The Anthropocene: Politik—Economics—Society—Science 12, DOI 10.1007/978-3-319-49803-4_4

These are examples of the killers' attempts to dehumanize their victims thus rendering it easy and appropriate to treat them in inhumane ways without any guilty conscience. By cutting up Miriam's father and scattering pieces of his flesh around so that they looked 'like the flesh of a goat', the killers seem to be in effect relegating his status to that of a goat and in the process anesthetizing themselves from the effects of the act of killing a fellow human being. By tying a dog to the back of Grace's father and forcing the dog to maul him to death, the killers seem to be making a symbolic statement about Grace's father being unworthy of human treatment.

Dehumanization has been used as an accompaniment for discrimination and atrocity throughout history. In his examination of the psychology of evil, seeking to understand why good people do evil, the psychologist Zimbardo (2007) in a sense blurs the line between good and evil, and argues that 'the barrier between good and evil is permeable and nebulous' (Zimbardo 2007: 2). Zimbardo emphasizes the boundless capacity of every state and person to commit evil, and traces the systematic murder of over 50 million people beginning with the 1915 Ottoman Turks killing of 1.5 million Armenians, through the Communist Khmer Rouge regime murder of 1.7 million people in Cambodia, to the 2006 genocide in Darfur, Sudan (Zimbardo 2007: 12). The killing of these groups of people is made psychologically acceptable through the process of dehumanization, rendering them as evil, morally inferior, less than human. 'War engenders cruelty and barbaric behavior against anyone considered the Enemy, as the dehumanized, demonic Other' (Zimbardo 2007: 17).

MacNair (2003: 2–3) refers to this tactic as 'semantic dehumanization', arguing that the words that describe an object, rather than the inherent nature of that object, determine one's perception of the object. The resultant 'linguistic warfare' has been used to facilitate violence against certain groups of people. By referring to people as 'deficient humans, nonhumans, nonpersons, animals, parasites, diseases, inanimate objects or waste products', violent acts against these groups of people becomes justified (MacNair 2003: 2). The tactic of semantic dehumanization made the extermination of the Jews by the Nazi regime possible and easy by referring to and perceiving the Jews as a disease, and the 1994 Rwandan genocide against the Tutsi by the Hutus by referring to and conceiving of the Tutsi as 'cockroaches' (Zimbardo 2007: 14).

And for what purpose? Why will human beings want to inflict such pain and horror on fellow human beings? Scarry (1985) argues that the intensity and absorbed manner of inflicting pain in torture signifies a deeper and far reaching goal; that of entrenching power. Scarry (1985: 27–28) describes the process by which this pain is translated into power:

> The physical pain is so incontestably real that it seems to confer its quality of "incontestable reality" on that power that has brought it into being… First, pain is inflicted on a person in ever-intensifying ways. Second, the pain, continually amplified within the person's body, is also amplified in the sense that it is objectified, made visible to those outside the person's body. Third, the objectified pain is denied as pain and read as power, a translation made possible by the obsessive mediation of agency.

Scarry (1985: 28) argues that what is in effect produced in this translation is 'a fantastic illusion of power'. It is not real. Scarry concludes that 'torture is a grotesque piece of compensatory drama'. For the participants who watched their loved ones tortured and killed in the atrocities of the war in South Sudan, the pain inflicted on the loved one's body converted into deep heart-felt pain for the survivors as expressed by Miriam in her cry:

> *I say... it is very painful. When I'm sleeping I just think in my mind ... how long will the Arab kill others like this? They get somebody and just kill and then they throw like this... They don't have any pain, to see that it is human being!* [With deep feeling of pain in her voice].[4]

The intensity of this pain translates into the illusionary power (Scarry 1985) felt by the perpetrators, whose domination leads the survivors to flee for safety. In making the pain and torture inflicted on their victims visible to the survivors, the perpetrators succeed in their mission of instilling fear and dread that causes the survivors to flee.

4.1.2 *Security:* 'No Rest'

One of the most common experiences among the refugees interviewed was the loss of security. Living in constant fear and not knowing what would happen next wore down on these survivors and was the main reason why they had fled to the camp. Refugees from the Nuba Mountains in South Kordofan especially expressed the deep, constant anxiety in which they lived as bombs from antonovs[5] were regularly thrown in the area, forcing the residents to flee to the mountains every day seeking refuge. As such, they experienced 'no rest' as Tahir, a 27 year-old man from the Nuba community expressed.[6]

Sometimes the very government soldiers from whom the survivors expect protection against attacks are the ones whom the participants blame for perpetrating the violence, as in the case of Patrick, a 40 year-old man from the Murle community.[7] Patrick described how he was beaten up by government soldiers and eventually decided to run. There has been an increase in attention to this feature of wars in which the government or the state turns against civilians, its own people, in recent decades, following the end of the Cold War (Paulson 2003). The civilian targets of these wars tend to be

---

[4]Interview with Miriam on 13 July 2013. See Appendix 4.1.

[5]An antonov is a Russian-made cargo plane converted into a crude bomber and used by the Sudan Armed Forces (SAF) in South Kordofan as a tool for civilian destruction and terror. The plane is not designed for use as an attack aircraft and has no bomb sighting mechanisms, allows no military purposeful aerial targeting, and is used for indiscriminate aerial bombardment, wreaking havoc in the lives of the civilians (McConnell 2013).

[6]Interview with Tahir on 4 July 2013. See Appendix 4.1.

[7]Interview with Patrick on 15 and 16 July 2013. See Appendix 4.1.

> … both poor and from a minority group, having few or no allies either in their home country or abroad… A key strategic goal in this type of warfare is to create terror among the targeted civilian population (Paulson 2003: 111).

In some instances, the violence that led the participants to flee for refuge is intertribal, especially as a result of cattle rustling between different tribes. Hiba,[8] a 30 year-old Nuer woman, related how 'some unknown people' came at night and killed people in her village, including her husband, destroyed property and took away cattle, forcing her and other survivors to flee for refuge. Patrick, a 40 year old from the Murle community, describes a similar scenario:

> *And my children ran to the bush where they went to hide ... And my wife was pregnant, then she delivered in the bush. It was during the fight. Then the following day I ran to bring them to the town. Then there had been a lot of murder, and some killing and harassment ... Yeah, I'm also traumatized. Yeah, because we are affected by this war, by seeing people being killed ... And people actually use the language of 'We want to wipe out Murle', you know. ... if you are abused, and told, 'You are rebel, or you are worthless', you know ... you feel psychologically depressed and this is now another, this is psychological war now... Yeah, psychological war, to injure you.*[9]

The main reason the refugees have fled from their country of origin is the pursuit of physical security—now that they do not feel safe and protected in their own land, they run for refuge. They run in search of a place where they can be secure, with a buffer against attack and possible extermination. The extermination they fear is on two fronts. Firstly there is the physical extermination, death. They literally run for their lives. Secondly, they dread what Patrick referred to as 'psychological war, to injure you'. His people are abused by others and called 'worthless… thieves… rebels', and this threatens their essence, leaving them vulnerable. They run to preserve their essence. The semantic dehumanization (MacNair 2003: 2) that entails using dehumanizing labels to refer to, and conceive of, certain groups of people as nonhumans or deficient humans not only serves to justify and facilitate acts of violence against the group of people, but affects the victims too, badly hurting them psychologically and rendering them all the more vulnerable. In the case of participants like Patrick who related these experiences, the survivors had tended to internalize these labels and as a result experience considerable psychological distress.

To the extent that the referent of security is the individual and not the state, the human security paradigm, based on the two notions of 'freedom from fear' and 'freedom from want' (Hayes/Mason 2013: 4–5), offers some explanation to the security considerations that forced the participants of this study to flee from their country of origin. They fled to protect their human security.[10]

---

[8]Interview with Hiba on 5 July 2013. See Appendix 4.1.

[9]Interview with Patrick on 15 and 16 July 2013. See Appendix 4.1.

[10]The human security paradigm has been invoked by various authors (Kaldor 2007; Marlies 2008; United Nations Trust Fund for Human Security 2009; Hayes/Mason 2013) to explain how structural violence causes refugee and migrant flows.

4.1.3 Separation: 'I Have No One Else'

Separation is another overarching trait of the participants' experience. The war in South Sudan is notorious for tearing families apart. Often, the outbreak of violence has resulted in separation of family members, each having run their own way, and not being able to find each other. In explaining the circumstances that led them to come to the camp, Abit, a 35 year old man from the Dinka community, described how this separation came to be:

> *So ... you run, you don't see your father even your mother ... You don't see anything ... I have no one else.*[11]

One of the most common features of this trait is children separated from their parents. Many survivors described how they were separated from their parents in their childhood and still do not know where their parents are to date. Joyce, a 40 year old woman from the Dinka community, was a recent arrival at the camp's Reception Centre and described her painful experience of being separated from her children:

> *I came with the children. I came here with four children, and some children went to play, and then we were attacked when two children were not around, so I didn't find them. Is there anywhere I can find those children? I need to bring them back here in this camp ...: I am now weak because my two children are not there and my younger child in now sick. Now I'm confused, I can't even tell this from that.*[12]

As a result of this separation, loneliness and loss, there is a disruption of the development of 'a cohesive self-structure'[13] which consists of an integration of one's sense of identity, value, meaning, and permanence, and an ability to accomplish one's goals without being rejected or isolated by loved ones and other important groups of people. This self-structure provides a sense of stability and permanence, and can maintain a sense of consistency even under threatening conditions. The self-structure and sense of permanence can be completely shattered by traumatic experiences, as appears to have happened in the case of the survivors (Baker/Baker 1987; White/Weiner 1986).

The separation and loss leads to a sense of loneliness that is described by the participants, such as Amuka, a 35 year old Dinka woman described:

> *And now, I came here without father, mother, no husband. When we arrived here, I looked for a husband, and I found one. After I gave birth to two children, the husband died. Now I'm remaining, lonely... before you came here, no one has ever visited me. I'm just here lonely, and staying here with the children, even no one realises that this woman is suffering from this and that.*[14]

---

[11]Interview with Abit on 2 July 2013. See Appendix 4.1.

[12]Interview with Joyce on 9 July 2013. See Appendix 4.1.

[13]The concept of a 'cohesive self-structure' is derived from Heinz Kohut's Self-Psychology model, especially as presented in his two famous works, *The Analysis of the Self* and *The Restoration of the Self*.

[14]Interview with Amuka on 3 July 2013. See Appendix 4.1.

Herman underlines the sense of disconnection that survivors of traumatic events feel, once all that they believed in, and that gave meaning to their lives, seems to have been shattered:

> Traumatic events have primary effects not only on the psychological structures of the self but also on the systems of attachment and meaning that link individual and community… Traumatized people feel utterly abandoned, utterly alone, cast out of the human and divine systems of care and protection that sustain life. Thereafter, a sense of alienation, of disconnection, pervades every relationship, from the most intimate familial bonds to the most abstract affiliations of community and religion (Herman 1997: 51–52).

The separation from loved ones and the uncertainty of ever seeing them again is comparable to the disappearances of political dissidents in Argentina and Colombia, which Taussig (1992: 19–20) says 'creates a new circle to Dante's hell in that it combines the terrible fact of loss with the ever-present hope that the disappeared will tomorrow, the next day … re-emerge.' Since 1977, the *Madres de Plaza de Mayo*, a social movement of 'Mothers of the Disappeared' in Argentina has been meeting weekly to protest the disappearance of an estimated 30,000 Argentines that occurred during Argentina's 'dirty war' (Bosco 2004). During this war, members of the Argentine security forces kidnapped, illegally detained, tortured and killed the victims (Bosco 2004: 383). Of particular concern to the *madres* is the fact that their sons and daughters simply disappeared and were never seen again. Some of the *madres*, in their protest, have found a way to publicly represent this disappearance and reject any form of consolation by representing themselves as 'perpetually pregnant, claiming that their sons and daughters are not dead, but rather still live inside their bodies, in their wombs…' (Bosco 2004: 392). This extreme form of representation by the *madres* of their loss underlines the problematic and traumatic ways in which separation and disappearance, apart from death, affects the survivor.

In other instances, there is certainty that the loved ones have died hence the separation is more permanent. Participants talked of having lost their loved ones in death, and in most cases, the killers are not identified specifically. The deaths are mostly described in the passive voice as shown in the italicized phrases in the following participants' words:

> Abit: '… may be *you lost* your parents, all of them.'[15]
> Pubudu: '… even my parents, my father and my mother… *they have gone.*'[16]
> Rachel: 'So my husband *was killed.*'[17]

[15]Interview with Abit on 2 July 2013. See Appendix 4.1.

[16]Interview with Pubudu on 5 July 2013. See Appendix 4.1.

[17]Interview with Rachel on 9 July 2013. See Appendix 4.1.

These participants do not say who killed their loved ones. In some instances, the participants report that 'some unknown people' came at night and attacked them, and they could not see the attackers clearly, as in the case of Hiba.[18] The enemy or perpetrator in the incidents described seems faceless and not clearly identifiable.

This facelessness of the perpetrator may well be either illusory or real, but either way serves the purpose of obliterating the participants' memory of the killing of loved ones. If one cannot assign a face or a particular identity to the person who committed the act, then one will not have to deal with the deep sense of loss the perpetrator has caused, the need for truth and justice, and the resultant realization of one's helplessness in doing anything about the act. If one sees the act of the loved one being killed as an occurrence that happened and not a deed that was done, then they might be better placed to let the matter rest and move on as it were. The perception of the other as faceless and unidentifiable then becomes more of a self-preservation measure for the survivor. This could be the veiled reasoning behind the facelessness of the enemy and the passivity of voice describing the act.

Albert Bandura's concept of moral disengagement in the exercize of moral agency (Bandura et al. 1996) offers an explanation for the notion of the faceless other. From their study examining the structure and impact of moral disengagement Bandura and his colleagues found, among other aspects, that 'obscuring or distorting the agentive relationship between actions and the effects they cause' served to make detrimental behavior appear to have little consequence (Bandura et al. 1996: 364–365). Based on Bandura's theory of moral disengagement, MacNair (2003) discusses the related tactic of 'distancing' which involves creating a 'mental distance from the reality of what is happening—isolation from horror, a mental barrier' (MacNair 2003: 3–4). The two theories explain how a perpetrator unflinchingly inflicts violence. In the case of the survivor of the violence, the reluctance or inability to assign an identity and agency to the perpetrator could be a form of mental distancing; a form of bulwark against the horror and sorrow resulting from the death of loved ones.

4.2 Long Journey Fleeing Attack

4.2.1 The Trek to Safety: 'Those Who Walked Far'

The survivors repeatedly related how they and their families had walked for long distances on foot in search of refuge. In these long journeys, there was scarcity of basic necessities such as food and water, as Fazila, a 21 year old woman from the Nuba community expressed:

[18]Interview with Hiba on 5 July 2013. See Appendix 4.1.

It was actually very difficult for us, especially because we were young by then. Walking without...water. We could sometimes get water from the river, but we really suffered so much. We could not get food. Our stepmother managed to escape with very little food. So it got finished, and we were actually crying, crying every day... So we went to Kauda, footing.[19] *We were footing. Three days, and three nights, no food, no water.*[20]

In addition, a number of survivors wanted to demonstrate the effect this walking for long distances had on their feet to date. Amuka, insisted that I look at her feet to see the damage done to them, 14 years on:

Yeah, I passed there footing alone, and still, my feet became, just look... [showing me her worn feet.][21]

Kerieme talked of having lost all his possessions, but then being able to purchase one extremely treasured pair of sandals that he used while walking to seek refuge:

I bought these [showing me the sandals on his feet] *in order that, I don't know whether I will get money again to buy something. I bought these because they might stay for long time....*[22]

From the interviews, a relationship of the survivors' difficult experiences to (their) feet emerged. It appears the participants' feet are a symbol that bears testimony to what the refugees have been through. The feet are the lowest point of the human's physical being. It is the feet that do the 'dirty work' of walking around, getting us where we want to go, and are constantly in touch with the ground. For the participants, the effects of the journey fleeing attack had affected their whole being, reaching to their utmost lowest levels, their feet. The effect could not go lower than that.

The feet bear the toll of the experience of the escape. The symbol is visible and telling, and serves as a constant reminder of what took place. Consequently, the feet and the journey they symbolize serve as a point of identity for the refugees. It places them apart from the rest of humanity, which has not had this experience. Many of them have encountered the story of 'The Lost Boys', a renowned group of young boys who fled South Sudan via Ethiopia and arrived in Kakuma in 1992. Some of 'The Lost Boys' are in Kakuma to date.[23] This group gained an identity of their own which is acclaimed the world over. A UNICEF (1996) report holds:

Among these were at least 20,000 children, mostly boys, between 7 and 17 years of age who were separated from their families. These 'lost boys' of the Sudan trekked enormous distances over a vast unforgiving wilderness, seeking refuge from the fighting. Hungry

[19]'Footing' is a terminology derived from the word 'foot' and used to mean walking for long distances. The term, a result of the corruption of the English language as spoken in many parts of East Africa, is in common usage and appears several times in the interviews.

[20]Interview with Fazila on 5 July 2013. See Appendix 4.1.

[21]Interview with Amuka on 3 July 2013. See Appendix 4.1.

[22]Interview with Kerieme on 4 July 2013. See Appendix 4.1.

[23]Atem, Abit, and Okot, participants in the interviews, were among The Lost Boys who arrived in Kakuma in 1992.

> frightened and weakened by sleeplessness and disease, they crossed from the Sudan into Ethiopia and back, with many dying along the way…The survivors who reached the camps in Ethiopia started to lead a relatively peaceful life. But it was not to last. This relative security was shattered again late in 1991 when fighting erupted around them, and they and children from other camps were on the move once more, eventually heading for Kenya.

The refugees in Kakuma whom I interviewed crave a similar identity, a grounding of their distinctiveness, especially in the face of so much disruption from their normal cultural practices and source of identity. In a sense they feel 'lost' in the camp. They would be 'Those who walked far'.

In her book *Identity and Power in Narratives of Displacement*, Powell (2015) provides a critique of the proclaimed identity of the 'The Lost Boys' and argues that it has been constructed to meet a particular need in the humanitarian discourse. The story of 'The Lost Boys' Powell (2015: 105) argues, is aimed at eliciting varying emotions in the people that encounter it, encouraging them to donate to the cause, while in fact it obscures the political situation that rendered the boys 'lost' and displaced in the first place, and does not offer any sustainable means of dealing with systematic violence. The story that creates this identity is itself problematic, as Powell argues, tracing its formation through the words of some of the 'Lost Boys' now living in the U.S. They formed these stories so that they could leave the refugee camps, telling what the sympathetic wanted, adding embellishments to the stories and making them as evocative as possible (Powell 2015: 112–113).

It is the story, not the actual happenings, or the causes thereof, that is the major concern in this case. The story is thus seen as a lifeline and the gateway to opportunities beyond the camp. How well and consistently a person can tell his or her story then becomes the determinant of such opportunities as resettlement or further studies. Fazila, a participant who had won a scholarship for further studies in Canada, described the scrupulous process of the interviews she and others had to go through, and emphasized the importance of consistency in the story one told during the interview:

> *So the first interview they take away some [people], second, up to the third. The third is the oral interview, they ask you the reasons why you fled your country, you know, and initially they did ask us to write the story. Autobiography. Why we left our country, and may be the reasons, the experiences we are facing here, and all that. So in the final one, which is oral, they ask us the same questions, they'd asked us when we were filling the form. So while we write in the first interview, the experiences that compelled us to flee from our country, the last interview they ask us to say them orally. So when your story differs from what you said, that is when now they will think you are lying. Because what you are not lying about, you can't lie, I mean you can't differentiate…Yeah, you may forget. So that's why many people mess… You can't know about some people. They give stories that are not true…. So when your story is differing, may be the time,… may be differing with the one you just told them, they know that you are lying. So your story should be in line with what you have just written. You should not divert even a little.*[24]

[24]Interview with Fazila on 5 July 2013. See Appendix 4.1.

Fazila's explanation, and particularly her emphasis on the importance of being consistent in the way one tells the story, underlines the discursive nature of the 'structure of the refugee' that Powell (2015: 113) refers to. In other words, the refugee has to be a certain way, his or her experiences need to comprise of certain evocative elements, and he or she needs to fulfill a pre-constructed image, and a disruption or diversion of this state of affairs shakes our experience of a stable and comfortable world.

Different scholars in the field of human rights have problematized the use of personal stories about poverty and survival to enhance descriptions of suffering and powerlessness (Kleinman/Kleinman 1996; Malkki 1998), arguing that such stories serve the purpose of justifying the claims for justice and human rights in the international arena. Butt (2002: 3) pointedly argues that these stories work as a 'rhetorical device' whose purpose is 'sustaining the illusions of a global morality' or 'human rights culture' which would not otherwise exist, without these stories. According to this argument, the stories, in effect, work to mask the actual absence of the voices of the suffering on the global stage.

This analysis of the way the stories are constructed and the purposes for which they are used is not to lead us to the dismissal of the accounts the survivors tell altogether, but rather to an awareness and a sensitivity to the dynamics that surround these accounts and how they might be interpreted. This awareness and sensitivity is seen to be crucial in considering ways of building sustainable peace, as will emerge in discussions in the next chapter.

4.3 Traumatic Experiences in the Camp

4.3.1 Pain in the Camp: 'Bad Blood'

> For sighing comes to me instead of food;
>   my groans pour out like water.
> What I feared has come upon me;
>   what I dreaded has happened to me.
> I have no peace, no quietness;
>   I have no rest, but only turmoil.
>   Job 3: 24–26

In the story quoted above, the Biblical character Job had gone through incredible suffering, having lost his sons and daughters and all that he owned within a matter of days, and eventually having painful sores all over his body. He penned the words quoted as he cursed the day of his birth. Like the Biblical Job, it seems sometimes the very threat from which the participants were attempting to escape when they fled their country of origin, follows them into the camp. Hiba, a mother of three, described her desperate situation when her children fell sick at the reception centre in the camp, and were running a very high fever at the time of the interview:

> *I went to the people here, when my children started getting sick two days ago. I went to the people at the clinic and told them these children are sick, may be they can help me. So these people were not willing to listen to me. They said they don't understand Arabic ... So I came back and I was sitting here. Again this morning I went and I started explaining to them that these children need fast medication, and these people, did not even care about what I was saying. And they said they were not listening to what I was saying. So I stayed there and when I saw there was no any assistance, I just decided to come here, and stay with these children, and just wait...*[25]

For Hiba, the place she has ran to for refuge from misery seems to be turning out to be a place of misery itself. While she is hopeful for relief from her troubles, Hiba finds herself in a precarious situation now with her two children urgently needing medication.

Sometimes the war is a direct cause of health problems such as people shot and maimed in the war, or, like in the case of Grace, who was raped by a soldier back in South Sudan. When tested for HIV/AIDS, she is diagnosed as having 'bad blood' as she puts it. Literally, her blood is contaminated so to say, as it is infected with the human immunodeficiency virus (HIV). Figuratively, she seems to imply that her blood, symbolizing the essence of her nature, is 'bad' in the sense that bad things 'naturally' happen to her. She represents many other refugees in the camp who feel misfortunes seem to readily fall on them.

Do misfortunes indeed readily fall on them? South Sudan has been at war for over five decades and the civilian population seems to have constantly borne the brunt of the war. In brooding over this question, sometimes the South Sudanese, who are deeply religious and most of whom adhere to the Christian faith, have attributed the seemingly wretched state of their land to the divine (Sudan Tribune 2012), and see the biblical words of Isaiah 18 as disturbingly referring to the land of South Sudan:

> Woe to the land of whirring wings
> along the rivers of Cush (the Nile)
> which sends envoys by sea
> in papyrus boats over the water.
> Go, swift messengers,
> to a people tall and smooth-skinned,
> To a people feared far and wide,
> an aggressive nation of strange speech,
> whose land is divided by rivers.
> All you people of the world,
> you who live on the earth,
> when a banner is raised on the mountains,
> you will see it,
> and when a trumpet sounds,
> you will hear it.

---

[25]Interview with Hiba on 5 July 2013. See Appendix 4.1.

> This is what the Lord says to me:
> "I will remain quiet and will look on
> from my dwelling-place,
> like shimmering heat in the sunshine,
> like a cloud of dew in the heat of harvest"
> (Isaiah 18:1–4).

Indeed, it does look like 'God remains quiet and looks on from [his] dwelling-place' and does not act on behalf of the people of this land, in spite of the atrocities they have experienced over decades. In Philip Caputo's novel *Acts of Faith* (2005: 3), the literary character Fitzhugh, a mixed-race Kenyan and former UN relief worker tries to explain the atrocious happenings in Africa in general and the Sudan in particular to the character Phyllis the American journalist with a rather fateful phrase: 'there is no difference between God and the Devil in Africa'. Is the state of affairs in South Sudan fateful?

While we may not be able to give reasons for the seemingly relentless atrocities in South Sudan, we can at least inquire into ways of avoiding similar suffering in the future, and consider possibilities of crafting sustainable peace.

4.3.2 *Scarcity:* 'Drying Up'

Kakuma refugee camp is situated in semi-arid land in Northwestern Kenya. It is hot, dry and dusty most of the year, and water is scarce. The heat and dryness seems to be reflected in the lives of the refugees and leaves them in what was described by participants as 'drying up':

'Drying up' here can be seen as a metaphor for lack of the vitality of life, both physically and emotionally. The scarcity and associated struggles tend to sap the survivors' energy, the very essence of their lives, and leave them dry. This was expressed by the participants, as the following excerpt from the interview with Zeneb, a 20 year old woman from the Dinka community, reveals:

> *I appreciate you... for asking me questions also, and for coming... because here in Kakuma, we are very dry...Yeah, we are drying up. This sun is very hot. So we appreciate the fact that you are here, and also burning together with us.*[26]

Reflecting on this dryness, I previously observed (Gitau 2013: 13) the following experiences of a resident new to the camp:

> At the border they boarded a UN vehicle that drove them the 100 kilometres to Kakuma Refugee Camp. Finally there was going to be relief! Their days of hunger, exhaustion, fear and hopelessness were coming to an end! …But as they drove on into the expansive camp, stretch after stretch of dry, rocky, empty, grey land spread before them. Where were the trees laden with fruit? Where was the milk, honey and gushes of fresh water? Where was food? And houses and children playing, and smiling people? Where?

[26]Interview with Zeneb on 3 July 2013. See Appendix 4.1.

> They finally got to the barbed wire-enclosed reception centre of the camp. Why did it look like a prison?

This aspect of the dryness of the camp is aptly captured by Agamben (1998: 170) in his conception of 'bare life' of the inhabitants of camps. Agamben conceives of a camp as a space of exception in which the normal juridical order is not in operation. Agamben's (1998: 174) description of camps spreads from his depiction of the Jewish concentration camps to embrace the camps constructed for various purposes in the post-World War II era, arguing that 'we find ourselves virtually in the presence of a camp every time such a structure [of the state of exception] is created'. With regard to 'bare life', Agamben (1998: 171) argues:

> Insofar as its inhabitants were stripped of every political status and wholly reduced to bare life, the camp was also the most absolute biopolitical space ever to have been realized, in which power confronts nothing but pure life, without any mediation.

The participants of the study may be categorized amongst those Agamben refers to as having 'bare life' in the sense that most of them fled their country of origin with barely anything other than their lives, as they fled attack and death. In the camp they find themselves in an uncertain situation, deprived of not only their material possessions and social connections that previously gave their lives meaning, but also their political status as citizens.

In this regard, the refugees fall in the category of people that Nash (2009: 1072–1079) refers to as 'un-citizens' in her discussion of the five types of citizens produced in the relationship between citizenship and human rights. 'Un-citizens' are 'mere humans' with no recognized political status and thus no state protection per se in the country they are living in. Humphrey (2002: 118–119) argues that the refugee,

> … the individual deprived of citizenship and dependent on the goodwill and moral responsibility of strangers (international community of states) has become the touchstone of global ethics. The refugee is par excellence the symbol of the cost of the international system of nation-states based on a hierarchy of exclusion.

In other words, by being deprived of citizenship, the refugee is deprived of human rights as well, and what he or she has left, in Agamben's (1998) words once again, is *homo sacer* (bare life). This bare life then, begs filling. Many of the survivors in the camp live in anticipation of a change of their circumstances, especially in terms of being considered for resettlement in a developed country, or 'going above',[27] as the participants called it.

[27]Interview with Juliet on 3 July 2013. See Appendix 4.1.

4.3.3 *Memories and Avoidance:* 'Dark Stone in My Stomach'

Some participants talked about their minds being preoccupied with the memories of the events surrounding the war back in their country, especially at night while in bed, and being very uncomfortable. In some rare cases, the participants used the words 'traumatized' and 'shocked' to express their feelings, like in the case of Riek, a 27 year old man from the Nuer community, describing the tragic death of his fiancée and his parents:

> *She just died during delivery...I feel traumatized. I was traumatized, I was shocked, a lot of things. It's just... negative all the time, what happened to me personally, what happened to my parents, so it is difficult... Sometime I do recall... being traumatized, when I'm in bed. ...Yeah when I'm in bed, I do recall what happened to me back home, ... I recall the trauma which happened when I was in my home country. And it was repeated year after year. I cannot forget ... I think, when I'm on my bed.*[28]

In some instances, there was awareness of feelings deeply buried within and not open to scrutiny. Okot, a 35 year old man from the Dinka community, expressed how he could not 'laugh like others' because there was 'something like a stone, dark stone in my stomach that somebody cannot see. But they see my teeth' and think 'I'm feeling okay'.[29]

In the revised Diagnostic and Statistical Manual of Mental Disorders (DSM-5) (1) (APA 2013), the diagnostic criteria for Post-Traumatic Stress Disorder (PTSD) include a history of exposure to a traumatic event that meets specific stipulations and symptoms from each of four symptom clusters: intrusion, avoidance, negative alterations in cognitions and mood, and alterations in arousal and reactivity. As noted in Riek's and Okot's relating of their experiences, the symptoms of intrusion, avoidance and negative alterations in cognition and mood were present among some of the participants. Intrusion symptoms involve recurrent, involuntary, and intrusive memories, traumatic nightmares and dreams. Riek remembered how his fiancée and unborn child died and thought about his experiences when he was in bed. He said he was 'traumatized' and 'cannot forget'. Okot said he avoided showing his true feelings and portrayed a seemingly happy disposition despite how he felt inside. The cases of Riek and Okot are examples of instances when participants showed symptoms specific to the PTSD criteria relating to memory and avoidance.

Banai et al. (2005: 225–228) explain what happens when people are traumatized as a result of mass violence. When people undergo traumatic experiences, they create psychological barriers against the painful experience, and may develop personality traits that lead them to avoid contact and deny the pain. The fatal, lost, far-away look observed amongst many of the participants may be said to conceal

[28]Interview with Riek on 11 July 2013. See Appendix 4.1.

[29]Interview with Okot on 2 July 2013. See Appendix 4.1.

the pain inside, but reveal this contact-shunning trait of those traumatized. This may also explain the avoidance of assigning agency or an identity to the people who did the killing, as observed in the previous section, in the use of passive voice to describe the deaths of loved ones, and attributing the killing to 'unknown people'.

Not in all cases was the pain avoided though. In some cases, the raw pain that came with the loss of loved ones was fresh and evident as in the case of Rachel who had recently lost a beloved husband in the war:

> *I feel a lot of pain, and I'm not happy in my life, because of losing my husband... I'm not happy.... I cannot feel again. I cannot have another husband .... Because my husband treated me nicely...I married in 2001, and he died in 2011. 10 years. I loved him a lot. He never beat me, he never insulted me, he just took care of me. Even all these dresses he bought for me* [she's dressed in a beautiful flowery African dress – 'kitenge'] ... *Nobody else is going to take care of me like that... I'm just thinking about the children... Sometimes I think too much I feel sick.... God knows now...*[30]

The pain she felt at her loss is clearly expressed here, but due to the disruption of their normal life and cultural practices, participants such as Rachel who feel the fresh pain of losing their loved ones are not able to undergo the normal grieving process.[31] This interrupted process of mourning can exacerbate the continuing effects of trauma and contribute to feelings of hopelessness and resignation expressed by some of the participants, as covered in the following section.

4.3.4 Resignation: 'Nothing'

A sense of powerlessness and resignation to the powers that be, tends to permeate through some of the interviews, and is here discussed in detail due to its significance in the lives of the survivors and its implications for peacebuilding. There is a particular powerlessness especially in relation to dependency on the UN in general and the UNHCR in particular for the participants' livelihood. Participants expressed that they would remain where the UNHCR was, or go where the UN took them. The two bodies, UNHCR and UN, were personified as it were, and a clear duality depicting 'they', the powerful and able (UNHCR, UN, God), versus 'we' the weak and vulnerable (refugees) was evident. Amuka expressed the personification this way:

> *There are two strong people here on earth. God, the Father, and UNHCR. UNHCR helps me by giving me shelter and food, and God helps me by giving me life, keeping me alive*

[30]Interview with Rachel on 9 July 2014. See Appendix 4.1.

[31]Traditionally, grieving and mourning among the South Sudanese is a community affair and is displayed openly and loudly. A widow is expected to mourn the death of her husband for at least 12 months, while the community takes care of her and her family (Sneesby et al. 2010). This grieving process is significantly disrupted by violence and resultant displacement of the survivors such as Rachel.

until this day. ... I am weak, I can't do any job, and I didn't go to school. I'm just there. Now it's just me, and UNHCR and God. We are the only three who live on this earth.[32]

This dependency that Amuka and other participants of the study expressed is aptly captured by Harrell-Bond (1986: 90–91) in her description of what it means to become a refugee:

> It should not be surprising that once refugees move under the aid umbrella their perceptions and behavior change. Numerous signals remind them that they are now being cared for by others. They are registered for assistance in a centre above which the UNHCR flag is flying. The sources of the food that they now eat are clearly marked on bags and tins. Even the colour of the vehicles in which they are transported inform them just who is now in charge of their salvation. They are told where to sleep, and with almost no advance notice, are ordered into a lorry and on a journey which may take many hours, taken to an unknown destination… Little wonder that refugees begin to refer to UNHCR as 'their mother and father'. … As UNHCR 'children', refugees have little choice but to completely surrender autonomy and freedom of action.

As with the case of the personal stories the refugees tell and their discursive nature, Butt (2002: 10) problematizes the issue of such dependency further by arguing that the image of the 'suffering stranger', or 'the poor', a category of people to which the refugees belong, has been constructed to legitimize a discourse of humanitarianism. Butt argues that the human rights culture needs this category of people to promote global claims of justice and human rights. Consequently, the poor learn to think in this same manner, from the paradigm of poverty, and 'embrace a collective identity based on notions of poverty' (Butt 2002: 15). The 'suffering stranger', so named to denote both this identity of poverty and his/her otherness or remoteness from his/her benefactors, is then

> …just such a child [of the pronouncer of this discourse]. She is a discursive construction that reduces global entanglements, and potentially rich human stories, to a moral model that allows for a sustained dependency between one group of people (i.e., those coded as needy) and another group of people (i.e., those coded as expert) (Butt 2002: 17).

In tracing the emergence of the status of 'refugee women' as a policy priority in UNHCR, Baines (2004: 9) also alludes to this creation of refugees as a category of people who are vulnerable and in need, but also 'located in safe humanitarian spaces in which UNHCR can enter and rescue the innocent'. This state of dependency leads to a kind of dead agency[33] for many of the participants, who see no need or have no motivation or ability to make decisions or do anything to affect their lives. Participants expressed a sense of having acquiesced with whatever may come their way. Expressions such as, 'Things just happened like that', as expressed

[32]Interview with Amuka on 3 July 2013. See Appendix 4.1.

[33]The concept of 'dead agency' here refers to the idea of being 'passive recipients of welfare-enhancing help' (Sen 1999: 189). The theme of agency in relation to coping strategies used by survivors in the camp, is discussed in the next chapter (Chap. 5).

by Zeneb,[34] were common. Chathuranjalee, a 26 year old woman from the Didinga community, similarly saw no part for herself to play in trying to improve her circumstances by going to school, as her words in the following excerpt reveal:

> *The husband says you just stay at home... Even if I'd like, what can I do. He says stay. If your husband says stay at home, wouldn't you stay?*[35]

When asked what services she thought would be helpful for her while in the camp, Chathuranjalee said:

> *I don't know* [resignedly]... *Here in Kakuma. I've told you those of us here in Kakuma, we just stay. There's nothing we are doing, nothing. But the problem as we stay here, the problem is food. Us we stay here... Nothing. You just get the ration, you make the food and eat, then we stay...I don't even know...Nothing. Even now as I speak to you, there's nothing... Here in Kakuma. I just stay, but if I want to go back, I just go back. (Pause). And if I want to stay, I stay. If I want to go back, I go back to Sudan.*[36]

These expressions suggest that according to these participants, their participation cannot contribute to anything worthy of note. The idea of 'just staying', denoting a non-participatory sense of existence rings through the interviews. There seems to be a certain deficiency in energy and ability to hold and sustain an opinion. As the author, Hosseini (2003: 311) so aptly says, 'Perspective was a luxury when your head was constantly buzzing with a swarm of demons.'

The experience of trauma refers to a paralysis or closing of the mind so that no more horror can enter. As MacNair (2003: 34) explains, one's mind and behavior are immobilized or numb, and the emotions are blocked, hence the constant expression of 'nothingness'. Herman (1997: 33) refers to psychological trauma as 'an affliction of the powerless'. In the case of these South Sudanese survivors, the sense of overwhelm and hence a feeling of inability to control their lives and what consequently happens to them is apparent.

In his unforgettable, shattering story of troubled Afghanistan, Hosseini (2003: 66–67) captures a similar sense of resignation and fatalism most poignantly in his account of the character Assef's rape of Hassan, a Hazara boy, as observed by Amir, and its uncanny comparison to the ritual yearly sacrifice of the lamb:

> Assef knelt behind Hassan, put his hands on Hassan's hips and lifted his bare buttocks. He kept one hand on Hassan's back and undid his own belt buckle with his free hand. He unzipped his jeans. Dropped his underwear. He positioned himself behind Hassan. Hassan didn't struggle. Didn't even whimper. He moved his head slightly and I caught a glimpse of his face. Saw the resignation in it. It was a look I had seen before. It was the look of the lamb... *The mullah finishes the prayer. Ameen. He picks up the kitchen knife with the long blade. The custom is to not let the sheep see the knife. Ali feeds the animal a cube of sugar – another custom, to make death sweeter. The sheep kicks, but not much. The mullah grabs it under its jaw and places the blade on its neck. Just a second before he slices the throat in one expert motion, I see the sheep's eyes. It is a look that will haunt my dreams for weeks.*

[34]Interview with Zeneb on 3 July 2013. See Appendix 4.1.

[35]Interview with Chathuranjalee on 17 July 2013. See Appendix 4.1.

[36]Interview with Chathuranjalee on 17 July 2013. See Appendix 4.1.

I don't know why I watch this yearly ritual in our backyard; my nightmares persist long after the bloodstains on the grass have faded. But I always watch. I watch because of that look of acceptance in the animal's eyes. Absurdly, I imagine the animal understands. I imagine the animal sees that its imminent demise is for a higher purpose. This is the look...

The look of desperation. Of acceptance. Of resignation. The look that seems to say, 'Let whatever happens happen. It does not matter.' As put by Zeneb in the interview, 'Things just happened like that'.[37] The progression of trauma that leads a person to such a state is as follows:

...the deepening of it manifested in a growing numbing of pain and painful emotions, followed by a loss of all vestiges of self-reliance, initiative, and agency. The empowerment to say "no" and to carry out self-defense was progressively lost. At a certain point, the traumatic closure reached a malignant state, with the blocking of all mental functions: cognition, registration of perceptions, recall, scanning, information processing in general, planning, and problem solving. Finally, just a vestige of these functions was retained, with some capacity for self-observation. If the traumatic process continued, all vitality was suppressed, and the individual succumbed to psychogenic death, with the heart stopping in diastole (Krystal 2004: 70).

Krystal (2004: 72) further gives an example of this progression of trauma by describing the Cambodian women, who during the genocidal attack, sometimes at the instant when their loved ones were about to be killed, developed a functional blindness which persisted for years, despite treatment.

The 'traumatic closure' Krystal described appears to have reached a perilous stage for Okot as he explains his inability to plan anything. The 'just staying' and the 'nothing' themes, signifying lack of a sense of anticipation or expectation is palpable as denoted in the following excerpt from the interview with Okot:

[After a pause]. *You know, here in the camp there are many things that are affecting us. When there is no way, you just keep quiet. You cannot think about it, you cannot talk about it, you can just keep quiet. That is what you conclude. Nothing happening on your planning, what you have planned or what you have decided to do ... you just, I just stay and forget everything...Yes, I just sit idly, and when I sit idly, I just look like I've forgotten.*[38]

Consequently then, a sense of despair and hopelessness ensues. There is a sense in which some refugees have lost hope of their lives and circumstances ever changing. The fact of having stayed in the camp since its establishment in 1992 without hope of things changing was expressed by a number of participants. Abit for example, who was one of the 'Lost Boys' who were the first residents in the camp said:

Me I'm still the same, that life. Nothing has changed in my life. My life is still the same as the day I came to Kenya.[39]

[37]Interview with Zeneb on 3 July 2013. See Appendix 4.1.

[38]Interview with Okot on 2 July 2013. See Appendix 4.1.

[39]Interview with Abit on 2 July 2013. See Appendix 4.1.

Joy, a 32 year old woman from the Acholi community, similarly described this disillusioned state in the following excerpt:

> *Psychologically we are not stable. For example if you reflect on the Sudanese community, you stay. Just stay. Some have forgotten what to do, some are frustrated, many have committed suicide ... For those who arrived in 1992, if you can still find them living up to this moment, then what is the hope? Also refugees are coming back from Sudan... If you look at the number of asylum seekers, a large population is coming from South Sudan.*[40]

Suleyman, a 27 year old from South Kordofan, summarized this sense of despair and hopelessness by saying:

> *... there was nothing at all. From the beginning, up to the end, there's nothing good, that I've seen in my life. And for all the entire people.*[41]

Faith in the systems and structures set up in the camp seems to be held in doubt too in some instances. Asked whether she was hopeful of assistance from the camp, Hiba expressed distrust saying:

> *I don't know. They are just putting the things in the computer. I don't know. They just gave me the card, and they told me to go.*[42]

Death, the survivors' own deaths, and not the death of loved ones, does not seem farfetched in these seemingly hopeless circumstances, as expressed by Dabor, a 46 year old woman from the Didinga community:

> *People are still fighting and funerals are full and increasing all the time ... I don't see. Now if all I can see is death, like the other day, after a short time, there's a funeral, someone has been killed in Sudan, on the road, do you see now? ... Those here get information, so and so has been killed, now that makes me fear, I might again come across something terrible.*[43]

Not only have some of the participants given up their grasp of life in the dependency and dead agency described above, they seem to have relinquished their right to keep alive against all odds. So much of some of these participants seems dead, that actual death would seem a mere extension of the life/death state they live in. Kristeva (1982: 4) describes this state of ultimate abjection, death, as being 'deprived of world', a state that 'no longer matches and therefore no longer signifies anything'. It is the 'nothing' state. Levi's (1959) concept of the *Muselmann*, in his autobiographical account of his time at Auschwitz, captures the 'nothing' state aptly. The term *Muselmann,* according to Levi, referred to the inmates of Auschwitz who, as a result of their intense suffering, lived in a life/death state, and

> ...drag[ged] themselves along in an opaque intimate solitude, and in solitude they die or disappear, without leaving a trace in anyone's memory ... non-men who march and labor in silence, the divine spark dead within them, already too empty to really suffer. One hesitates

---

[40]Interview with Joy on 16 July 2013. See Appendix 4.1.

[41]Interview with Suleyman on 10 July 2013. See Appendix 4.1.

[42]Interview with Hiba on 5 July 2013. See Appendix 4.1.

[43]Interview with Dabor on 16 July 2013. See Appendix 4.1.

to call them living; one hesitates to call their death death, in the face of which they have no fear, as they are too tired to understand (Levi 1959: 67–69).

Though there are exceptions to this state as will emerge in the discussion in the next chapter, for some of the participants whose experiences are related in this chapter, death seems to be the ultimate condition of the 'nothing' state.

This sense of powerlessness, resignation and disillusionment has ramifications for the work of peacebuilding. If the participants feel that they cannot contribute anything to improve their circumstances, are resigned as passive recipients to anything that is done for them, and have lost hope of circumstances improving anyway, and even in some instances are seemingly waiting for death, then they are unlikely to participate in peacebuilding activities geared to improve the situation that rendered them powerless in the first place. The likelihood of the recurrence of the cycle of events leading to violence, and need for refuge, intensifies.

4.3.5 *Gendered Contours:* 'He Took Me by Force'

Of particular note is the gendered ways in which the participants are impacted by the violence and resultant displacement into the refugee camp. Both men and women are impacted in differentiated and multifaceted ways that undermine their ability to negotiate the challenges of displacement. While female participants particularly expressed their vulnerability and ways in which they were affected, male participants did not readily express these effects, and only two aspects of the gendered ways in which men are impacted, the despondency resulting from the dependency on UNHCR for provisions and the inability to acquire dowry to marry according to their traditional custom, are discussed in this section.[44] Women participants discussed rape, domestic violence, unequal opportunities to education, wife inheritance, unwanted pregnancy and sexually-transmitted diseases among the issues that affected them.

Miriam expressed the insecurity young women face in the camp, for example the threat of rape, when they go out to try and collect firewood in the camp fields:

Maybe sometimes I may decide to go to Laga to collect a little firewood, then come back and cook. Maybe I don't know that you cannot trust people in Kakuma. So maybe sometimes I will just go to Laga and get people who will rape me... I don't know. That is why I fear.[45]

[44]A discussion of the reasons for this disparity, and a thorough consideration of the theme of gender in the context of mass violence, is beyond the scope of this book. While there has been a sustained focus on the impact of mass violence and displacement on female survivors, there exists a gap in research on ways in which male survivors are impacted.

[45]Interview with Miriam on 13 July 2013. See Appendix 4.1.

The threat of rape as a looming danger for the women in the camp was further expressed by Joy:

> *But you find such a thing still happens in the camp... as a single mother or a single girl. People are forcing you to have aah,* yaani *[like]... sex, they are defiling girls, they are raping women... You find women don't have a voice and that courage to report.*[46]

The legacy of rape committed during the war back in their country of origin continues to affect some of the survivors. Grace is a case in point. She described how she had been a victim of rape back in South Sudan and been forced to marry the perpetrator. As a result, she had contracted HIV/AIDS:

> *Just those issues of Sudan. You know there in Sudan earlier on I had another husband, who held me by force [raped me] as a result of the war... Yes. He took me by force, and I lived with him, until now when I had the children, the children cannot stay ... so the children died. Now I can't go back to Sudan. Because of those issues of war....my blood came out bad. That I have bad blood... Like HIV/AIDS.*[47]

In her presentation of a case study of survivors of sexual violence in South Sudan, D'Awol (2011: 53) discusses the pervasiveness of the violence during South Sudan's civil wars, and notes that it 'remains a terrible legacy of the wars' today. Women are at an increased risk for gender-based violence, including sexual violence, and the aggressors range from soldiers to the refugee or IDP men with them in the camp. Pittaway/Pittaway (2004) specifically discuss the case of refugee women in Kakuma, based on their research examining the prevalence of sexual and gender based violence amongst refugee women and the inadequacy of international interveners to protect the women. Pittaway/Pittaway (2004: 10) argue that the label 'Refugee Woman' renders the women in the camp vulnerable and exposed to more abuse, and restrains them from expressing their other identities.

The interconnection of conflict, mass violence and rape is evident from the above interview excerpts. As Hirschauer (2014: 235) argues in her discussion of the securitization of rape, the Bosnian war and Rwandan genocide propelled rape in war to the fore as a key security issue, with the first convictions of rape as a crime against humanity in the International Criminal Tribunal for the former Yugoslavia in relation to Bosnia, and rape as a crime of genocide in the International Criminal Tribunal for Rwanda. Hirschauer (2014: 186) notes:

> Yet, amid the most unimaginable, the anguish and the suffering of tens of thousands of rape and sexual violence survivors during both conflicts, something else happened. The suffering mattered. It was a shift, an un-licensing, an undoing of a status quo, endorsed for centuries. An unraveling of the unspoken; a new look at the customs, rules and the once so well-established and commonly understood narrative of war.

The recognition of rape as a war crime was a critical step toward understanding rape as violence, but as Copelon (1995) argues, the line between rape committed during wartime and rape committed at other times is not so sharp. Rape, in both war

---

46Interview with Joy on 16 July 2013. See Appendix 4.1.

47Interview with Grace on 17 July 2013. See Appendix 4.1.

and peace, needs to be recognized and addressed as a human rights issue (Richters 1998: 112; Fiske/Shackel 2014: 4190). Indeed, a sharp distinction between rape in war and rape in peace tends to diminish the import of rape as an egregious crime at all times and to put in jeopardy what happens after war is over: as points out:

When the ethnic war ceases or is forced back into the bottle, will the crimes against women matter? Will their suffering and struggles to survive be vindicated? Or will condemnation be limited to this seemingly exceptional case? (Copelon 1995: 199)

This is particularly true for participants like Grace who continue to experience the effects of rape while in the camp, having been infected with HIV/AIDS and losing her children at birth, as well as having to flee for safety in the camp. Her case is poignantly captured by Richters' (1998: 118) argument that the traumatic consequences of wartime rape are complex and multifaceted because:

> …in war, women often suffer multiple traumatization and rape trauma mixes with other traumas such as the loss of husbands, children, parents, relatives, homes, etc. What is experienced as the dominant trauma, and why that is the case, is often hard to detect and can vary in individuals and cultures.

In discussing the dynamics at play in the use of rape in wartime, Stefatos (2012) uses the case of the Greek Civil War of 1946 to 1949 to illustrate how the female body was in effect, through rape, being used to further political agenda. Stefatos (2012: 57) argues:

> Sexual violence in wartime is not simply attacking the female body; it is primarily intended to suffocate the political body. The legitimization of violence against women is primarily an exercise of political power … The target was not only the physical body but also the disintegration of the community and social chaos.

Rape has been a common act of war through the ages, in wars of all types—wars of religion, wars of revolution, wars on terror and wars of revenge (Brownmiller 1975). Brownmiller makes the point that 'rape is the quintessential act by which a male demonstrates to a female that she is conquered—vanquished—by his superior strength and power' and as such, it was used by the Germans and the Japanese during World War II to achieve their objective of 'total humiliation and destruction of "inferior peoples"' (p. 49). Baines (2004: 2) similarly argues that 'Women's bodies symbolize the markers of some imagined nation, and "intimate" violence is employed… to either eradicate or to create national boundaries and further political agendas'. The goal of rape is not only to attack and degrade the integrity and identity of the victim, but to dominate and dehumanize (Copelon 1995: 199–200). In the case of the participants of this study who talked about rape, it is not just a strategy that was used in the violence back in their country of origin, but its impact continues to be experienced in the camp.

The varied experiences of female survivors in situations of conflict and violence is further seen with regard to education opportunities in the camp. Even in situations where opportunity is seemingly given to all for access to education, women are in some ways rendered powerless to take advantage of these opportunities, as in the case expressed by Joy. Joy dropped out of school because she was unable to sit the required qualifying exams after a disruption in the camp that left her with no books or change of clothes, as she explained:

> *Yeah. So they said that we should sit for qualification, then when that incident happened I was somehow disorganized, having no books to revise, no clothes to change, also as a lady it was somehow difficult to cope with the situation having left with one set of clothes ... Then when others were sitting for the qualification, I did not even sit for the qualification.*[48]

In discussing the differentiated ways in which women experience the consequences of mass violence, Ni Aolain et al. (2011: 34) point to the 'unequal power relations' present in the cultural norms of the community, and how they 'translate into differential access to health resources, to education, to income, and to political voice'. In the case of Joy and others like her in the camp, being a woman meant that they could not access education opportunities provided in the camp in the same way as their male counterparts.

Another critical effect of the mass violence and displacement has been the disruption of the family system caused by death and separation, resulting in high numbers of widows or women separated from their husbands. Female participants especially expressed the difficulty they faced as a result of being separated from their husbands, as expressed by Rita, a 29 year old woman from South Kordofan, who had recently arrived in the camp:

> *I'm married but my husband I don't know where he is... My life is difficult because my husband, I don't know where he is. Life has become very difficult because my husband would help in each situation, difficult or easy...then my husband I don't know where he is. Life for me becomes very difficult, then I think a lot.*[49]

In addition, practices related to marriage have taken on a new bearing as a result of death and separation, as with the case of Rachel who was threatened with wife inheritance after her husband died in the army. Wife inheritance is a custom practiced traditionally in many communities in South Sudan, which sees a woman getting married to her husband's brother, once her husband dies. Rachel explained:

> *Now I'm 29.... So my husband was killed, and when I remained at home, I was being treated badly by the brother of my husband. Because we have that custom there, if the husband dies, he (the brother-in-law)) wants to take me to be his wife... So me I had an operation.... he (my husband) left me pregnant. I was about to deliver. I was very sad because he died, I never took care for myself... I delivered through an operation. And he (the brother-in-law) wanted me to be his wife. He even took my two children, the first two children of mine, he took them by force. But my father took them again from him.*[50]

With this disruption of the family system as they knew it before coming to the camp, women tend to take on new roles to survive, the situation in effect resulting in role reversal. Joy, for example, further explained the plight facing women of her

[48]Interview with Joy on 16 July 2013. See Appendix 4.1.

[49]Interview with Rita on 4 July 2013. See Appendix 4.1.

[50]Interview with Rachel on 9 July 2013. See Appendix 4.1.

community in the camp who turn to brewing illicit brew in order to fend for their families, because they 'have no other option'.

This situation of role reversal is related to the dependency on UNHCR for provision of basic necessities, and the survivors being forced into a life of inactivity. Male survivors are particularly affected by this state of dependency. In South Sudanese cultures, the man is supposed to go out and fend for his family while the wife stays at home and looks after the children. The dependency on UNHCR in the camp has changed this dynamic, and as expressed by Joy, has led men to tend to forfeit their responsibilities in taking care of their families:

> *In this camp, most men are irresponsible. ... They say, WFP is providing food...Yeah. The men here tell us... because all of us are having the same status, we get the same size of ration, we all depend on UNHCR... They say UNHCR and WFP...is providing food. To everyone. So we are equal. And they also say, each child comes with the budget. Because each child, after being delivered, is added to the ration in your card, and is entitled to the same ration size.*[51]

Not only do the men see no point, they also have no means of providing for their families in the camp. Pittaway (2013: 172) discusses the erosion of the culture and its resultant disruption of the order of life the refugees previously led:

> Men are not permitted to undertake their roles as providers, while women's traditional roles as mothers and wives are eaten away by conflict and the institutionalism of camp life. ...
>
> In these difficult situations, refugees suffer from serious challenges to their cultural heritage and their ability to maintain family and community life. They struggle to maintain their capacity to create a sustainable lifestyle for themselves and their families.

Another situation that has tended to affect male survivors in particular is with regard to marriage. The marriage institution as practiced traditionally in South Sudanese cultures has been greatly affected. For instance, through the breakdown and separation of families and loss of property, young men find it difficult to secure the dowry needed in order to marry, and gain the subsequent status in the community that comes with being married. Riek expressed how his fellow clansmen did not take him seriously because he had reached the age of marriage but had not yet got married, as a result of the tragedy that had struck his parents, wife-to-be and his unborn child.

These experiences illustrate a key consequence of the survivors' experiences of the war—the breakdown of their culture. The excerpts provide evidence that the experience of war and the resultant displacement into the camp translates into the destruction of the survivors' social capital: their capacities, networks, resources and relationships that previously worked for them.

[51]Interview with Joy on 16 July 2013. See Appendix 4.1.

4.4 Conclusion

The theme of dehumanization emerges as a critical issue for the participants, in relation to the torture and death of the participants' loved ones back in their country of origin. The loss of security is also an overarching condition that characterizes the participants' flight for refuge in the camp. Further, separation from loved ones emerges as another predominant trait, and is seen to result in loneliness and disrupt the participants' sense of identity, value and meaning.

In considering the participants' literal journey fleeing attack, their expressions of how they and their families walked for long distances in search of refuge predominates. The relationship the participants draw between their experiences and their feet, and ways in which the feet and the journey they symbolize serve as a point of identity resonates with the story of The Lost Boys.

Within the camp, the participants are seen to experience disease, scarcity, memories of traumatic experiences back in their country of origin, and resignation. Disease is seen as an example of the seemingly fateful circumstances of the survivors. A consideration of the theme of fate is seen to lead us to an inquiry into the ways of avoiding a repeat of what the participants have suffered and consider possibilities of crafting sustainable peace.

The notion of scarcity as expressed by the participants is captured by Agamben's (1998) concept of 'bare life' denoting a state in which the survivors are deprived of citizenship and other human rights, and left with a bare life that begs filling. Memories and avoidance, symptoms specific to the PTSD criteria portrayed by some of the participants, reveal the deep pain the participants conceal inside as a result of their traumatic experiences. Resignation, which is discussed in relation to the participants' dependency on the UN and the UNHCR, is seen to have ramifications for the work of peacebuilding.

Lastly, the gendered ways in which the participants are impacted by the violence and resultant displacement into the refugee camp complicate the participants' ability to negotiate the challenges of life in the camp and the path to peacebuilding. The threat of rape remains a looming danger for the women in the camp, and the consideration of rape in the context of mass violence as a separate issue from rape in peace time puts in jeopardy the treatment of rape as a grievous human rights violation at all times. The breakdown of the participants' culture, and in particular the disruption of the family system, leads to the destruction of the participants' social capital, rendering engagement in productive activities difficult.

As will emerge in the next chapter, there are exceptions to the seemingly desperate situations and reactions to the events of the conflict in South Sudan discussed in this chapter, and there are participants who appear to have negotiated the events in creative ways, sometimes through self-motivation, other times as a result of interventions received in the camp.

Appendix 4.1

Pseudonym	M/F	Ethnic group	Age	Duration of stay in the camp	Brief details	Date of interview
Miriam	F	Nuba	20	9 years	Fled South Kordofan when Arabs (North Sudanese) attacked and her father, uncle and other relatives were killed. Watched the Arabs kill her father and cut up his flesh into pieces. Other relatives joined her in 2013	13th July 2013
Grace	F	Acholi	40	14 years	Father and brother tortured and killed on being suspected to be traitors. Raped and forced into marriage by a soldier. Has given birth 14 times and only one child has survived. Also taking care of 10 of her deceased brothers' children. Was diagnosed HIV positive in the camp and resettlement process stalled. Cooks food for sale to supplement the ration in the camp	17th July 2013
Tahir	M	Nuba	25	1 month	Escaped war in South Kordofan. Family members were killed	4th July 2013
Amuka	F	Dinka	35	14 years	Walked to Kakuma, escaping both the war in South Sudan and an abusive husband. Married again in the camp and husband died. Lives with her two children in the camp	3rd July 2013
Patrick	M	Murle	40	5 months	People from the Nuer Community attacked his village and killed many people, his wife and children ran to the bush where his wife delivered their last child. SPLA soldiers attacked his village, many people were killed and he sustained injuries. Worked as a Livestock officer. In the Reconciliation committee between the Murle and the Nuer in the camp	15th and 16th July 2013

(continued)

(continued)

Pseudonym	M/F	Ethnic group	Age	Duration of stay in the camp	Brief details	Date of interview
Hiba	F	Nuer	30	2 months	Fled home in South Sudan when unknown people attacked and her husband and others were killed. Is in the camp with three children aged seven, three and one. The youngest two were running a very high fever at the time of the interview	5th July 2013
Abit	M	Dinka	35	21 years	Working as a volunteer in peacebuilding in the camp. Was sponsored by someone in Texas USA to go back to school from 2003 to 2006. Was among 'The Lost Boys'	2nd July 2013
Chathuranjalee	F	Didinga	26	6	Fled war between the North and the South, in which her parents were killed. Living in the camp with husband who works in the camp hospital and two little children, one in preschool in the camp	17th July 2013
Joyce	F	Dinka	40	4 months	Her village was attacked by the Nuer who came cattle raiding and her husband, father and mother were shot dead. Came with four children. Two children are still missing	9th July 2013
Joy	F	Acholi	32	12 years	Fled civil war in South Sudan and came to camp with cousin. Mother joined her in 2003. Was unable to complete secondary education in the camp. Case worker with LWF Peacebuilding unit. Has two children and is expecting a third in a month's time. Separated from her husband	16th July 2013
Suleyman	M	Nuba	27	4 years	Fled discrimination in South Kordofan and joined his brother in the camp. Gave a	10th July 2013

(continued)

(continued)

Pseudonym	M/F	Ethnic group	Age	Duration of stay in the camp	Brief details	Date of interview
					brief history of the different civil wars and peace attempts between the South and the North. Has received counselling services and training from JRS	
Rita	F	Nuba	29	1 month	Came to the camp as a result of war in South Kordofan. Father was killed and family dispersed. She does not know where her husband is. Living with her three year-old son, and is pregnant	4th July 2013
Dabor	F	Didinga	46	20 years	Escaped war between the North and the South. Parents and husband died in the war. Feared her children would be recruited as child soldiers and fled. Remarried in Kakuma, got two other children and second husband also died in the war when he went back to fight. Was working as a midwife in Kakuma hospital but lost her job in 1999. Cooks doughnuts to sell in the camp	16th July 2013
Pubudu	M	Nuer	20	4 years	Came to the camp when uniformed people attacked their village and family dispersed. Does not know where family members are	5th July 2013
Rachel	F	Nuer	29	3 months	Her husband was an SPLA soldier and was killed in the war in South Sudan. Was threatened with wife inheritance by the brother of her the husband, who also abused her. Escaped the abuse. Has five children but living with three in the camp, while two are with her father in South Sudan. Still suffering pain from wounds sustained during delivery, and fear of her husband's brother. Can speak seven South Sudanese languages and helps camp officials with interpretation	9th July 2013

(continued)

(continued)

Pseudonym	M/F	Ethnic group	Age	Duration of stay in the camp	Brief details	Date of interview
Kerieme	M	Nuba	20	1 month	At the Reception Centre waiting to be settled in the Camp. Came all alone to Kakuma from Yida IDP camp and does not know where other family members are	4th July
Fazila	F	Nuba	21	14 years	Family escaped due to the war between South Sudan and Arabs in 1999. Came to the camp with step-mother and two siblings. Father an SPLA. Mother joined them in the camp in 2012. Has won scholarship and is preparing to go to University in Canada in August	5th July 2013
Zeneb	F	Dinka	20	20 years	Born in the camp. Father went back to South Sudan in 1996 and was short dead. Moved to Nairobi with mother in 2003 to attend school. Mother died in 2010 as a result of wounds sustained in the post-election violence in Kenya in 2008. Working as an incentive case worker with Peacebuilding unit of LWF	3rd July 2013
Juliet	F	Dinka	23	21 years	Came to the camp with mother after they were attacked by a neighbouring tribe and the father was shot dead back in South Sudan. Went back to South Sudan in 2007 but came back to the camp after receiving no help there. Husband died in an accident. Lives with her two children, mother and sister	3rd July
Okot	M	Dinka	33	21 years	Was teaching in a Special Needs nursery school in the camp but was retrenched in 2011. Doing a Laboratory course in the Camp hospital. Was among 'The Lost Boys'	2nd July 2013

(continued)

(continued)

Pseudonym	M/F	Ethnic group	Age	Duration of stay in the camp	Brief details	Date of interview
Riek	M	Nuer	27	8 years	Escaped due to insecurity after his parents, fiancée and unborn child died. Has taken advantage of different education opportunities in the camp. Works as a community leader. Involved in reconciliation efforts between the Nuer and the Murle tribes in the camp	8th July 2013

References

Agamben, G. (1998). *Homo Sacer: Sovereign Power and Bare Life*. Stanford: Stanford University Press.

Baines, E.K. (2004). *Vulnerable Bodies: Gender, the UN and the Global Refugee Crisis.* Aldershot: Ashgate.

Baker, H.S. & Baker, M.N. (1987). 'Heinz Kohut's Self Psychology: An Overview'. In *The American Journal of Psychiatry,* Vol. 144, No. 1, pp. 1–9.

Bandura, A., Barbaranelli, G., Caprara, V. & Pastorelli, C. (1996). 'Mechanisms of Moral Disengagement in the Exercise of Moral Agency'. In *Journal of Personality and Social Psychology*, Vol. 71, No. 2, pp. 364–374.

Bosco, F. (2004). 'Human Rights Politics and Scaled Performances of Memory: Conflicts among the Madres de Plaza de Mayo in Argentina'. In *Social and Cultural Geography*, Vol. 5, No. 3, pp. 381–402.

Brownmiller, S. (1975). *Against Our Will: Men, Women and Rape*. New York: Simon and Schuster.

Butt, L. (2002). 'The Suffering Stranger: Medical Anthropology and International Morality'. In *Medical Anthropology,* Vol. 21, No. 1, pp. 1–24.

Caputo, P. (2005). *Acts of Faith.* New York: Vintage Books.

Copelon, R. (1995). 'Gendered War Crimes: Reconceptualizing Rape in Time of War'. In Peters, J. & Wolper, A. (Eds.) *Women's Rights: International Feminist Perspectives.* New York: Routledge, pp. 197–214.

D'Awol, A.M. (2011). '*Sibu ana, sibu ana* ('leave me, leave me')': Survivors of Sexual Violence in South Sudan'. In Bubenzer, F. & Stern, O. (Eds.) *Hope, Pain & Patience: The Lives of Women in South Sudan.* Wynberg: Institute for Justice and Reconciliation.

Fiske, L. & Shackel, R. (2014). 'Ending Rape in War: How Far Have We Come?' In *Cosmopolitan Civil Societies: An Interdisciplinary Journal*, Vol. 6, No. 3, pp. 4183–4193.

Gitau, L. (2013) 'Where is Hope? Rakela in Kakuma', *PeaceWrites*, 2. Sydney: Centre for Peace and Conflict Studies, University of Sydney, pp. 13–14.

Harrell-Bond, B.E. (1986). *Imposing Aid: Emergency Assistance to Refugees.* Oxford: Oxford University Press.

Hayes, A. & Mason, R. (2013). 'Security in Twenty-first Century Societies'. In Steiner, N., Mason, R. & Hayes, A. (Eds.) *Migration and Insecurity: Citizenship and Social Inclusion in a Transnational Era.* London: Routledge, pp. 3–16.

Herman, J. (1997). *Trauma and Recovery*. New York: Basic Books.

Humphrey, M. (2002). 'Humanitarianism, Terrorism and the Transnational Border'. *Social Analysis,* Vol. 46, No. 1, pp. 117–122.

Hirschauer, S. (2014). *The Securitization of Rape: Women, War and Sexual Violence*. London: Palgrave Macmillan.

Hosseini, K. (2003). *The Kite Runner*. London: Bloomsbury.

Kleinman, A. & Kleinman, J. (1996). 'The Appeal of experience, the dismay of images: Cultural appropriations of suffering in our times'. *Daedalus,* Vol. 125, No. 1, pp. 1–23.

Kristeva, J. (1982). *Powers of Horror: An Essay on Abjection.* New York: Columbia University Press.

Krystal, H. (2004). 'Resilience: Accommodation and Recovery'. In Knafo, D. (Ed.) *Living With Terror, Working With Trauma: A Clinician's Handbook.* Lanham: Jason Aronson, pp. 67–82.

Levi, P. (1959). *If This Is A Man.* London: Orion Press Limited.

MacNair, R. (2003). *The Psychology of Peace: An Introduction*. Wesport, CT: Praeger.

Malkki, L. (1998). 'Things to Come: Internationalism and Global Solidarities in the late 1990s'. *Public Culture,* Vol. 10. No. 2, pp. 431–442.

Nash, K. (2009). 'Between Citizenship and Human Rights'. *Sociology,* Vol. 43. No. 6, pp. 1067–2083.

Ni Aolain, F., Haynes, D.F. & Cahn, N. (2011). *On the Frontlines: Gender, War, and Post-Conflict Process.* Oxford: Oxford University Press.

Paulson, D.S. (2003). 'War and Refugee Suffering'. In Krippner, S. & McIntyre, T.M. (Eds.) *The Psychological Impact of War Trauma on Civilians: An International Perspective*. London: Praeger, pp. 111–122.

Pittaway, E. & Pittaway, E. (2004). '"Refugee Woman": A Dangerous Label: Opening a Discussion on the Role of Identity and Intersectional Oppression in the Failure of the International Refugee Protection Regime for Refugee Women'. In *Australian Journal of Human Rights*, Vol. 20, pp. 1–13.

Pittaway, E. (2013). 'Citizens of Nowhere: Refugees, Integration Criteria and Social Inclusion.' In Steiner, N., Mason, R. & Hayes, A. (Eds.) *Migration and Insecurity: Citizenship and Social Inclusion in a Transnational Era*. London: Routledge, pp. 169–187.

Powell, K. (2015). *Identity and Power in Narratives of Displacement*. New York: Routledge.

Richters, A. (1998). 'Sexual Violence in Wartime: Psychosociacultural Wounds and Healing Processes: the Example of the Former Yugoslavia'. In Bracken, P.J. & Petty, C. (Eds.) *Rethinking the Trauma of War.* London: Free Association Books, pp. 112–127.

Scarry, E. (1985). *The Body in Pain: The Making and Unmaking of the World.* Oxford: Oxford University Press.

Sen, A. (1999). *Development as Freedom*. Oxford: Oxford University Press.

Sneesby, L., Satchell, R., Good, P. & van der Riet, P. (2010). 'Death and Dying in Australia: Perceptions of a Sudanese Community'. Retrieved 29 June 2015 from: http://journals.sfu.ca/hneh/index.php/hneh/article/viewFile/62/53.

Stefatos, K. (2012). 'The Victimization of the Body and the Body Politic during the Greek Civil War, 1946–49'. In Branche, R. & Virgili, F. (Eds.) *Rape in Wartime*. New York: Palgrave Macmillan.

Sudan Tribune (2012). 'South Sudanese Christians plan "prophesied" pilgrimage to Israel'. Retrieved 20 July 2015 from: http://www.sudantribune.com/spip.php?article41707.

Taussig, M. (1992). *The Nervous System*. London: Routledge.

UNICEF (1996). 'The Lost Boys of the Sudan'. Retrieved 9 May 2015 from: http://www.unicef.org/sowc96/closboys.htm.

White, M.T., Weiner, M.B. (1986). *The Theory and Practice of Self Psychology*. New York: Brunner/Mazel Publishers.

Zimbardo, P. (2007). *The Lucifer Effect: Understanding How Good People Turn Evil.* New York: Random House.

Chapter 5
Strong at the Broken Places: Coping with Traumatic Experiences

> *The world breaks everyone, and afterward, some are strong at the broken places.*
>
> Ernest Hemingway, *A Farewell to Arms*, 1929

5.1 Basic Necessities: '*The Ration Card*'

The refugees first receive the basic needs of food, shelter, protection and recognition as refugees when they arrive in Kakuma. Not only have the refugees suffered from scarcity of basic necessities of food and water during their long journey fleeing attack, but they have been uprooted from their homes of origin, leaving them in an unfamiliar and lost state, hence necessitating the assigning of the refugee status. The ration card received from UNHCR serves as an identity and a key to receiving the basic necessities in the camp, as Chriz, a 23 year old man from South Kordofan pointed out:

> *Yeah, first time we arrived here, we were given the ration cards, which assist us to get very many services like food, water and housing. If we are not given the ration card, then we are not refugees, that's why the first thing we were to get is the ration card, and it assisted us in very many ways.*[1]

A number of the participants wore the UNHCR ration card on a string around their necks, which seemed to portray it as some kind of icon on which their lives hang.

The UNHCR, also known as the UN Refugee Agency, was established in 1950 and mandated by the UN to support and protect refugees (UNHCR 2015). The parallel 1951 Convention relating to the Status of Refugees is the key legal document that defines who is a refugee, their rights and the legal obligations of states (UNHCR 2001). Article 1 of the Convention defines a refugee as:

> a person who is outside his/her country of nationality or habitual residence; has a well-founded fear of persecution because of his/her race, religion, nationality, membership in a particular social group or political opinion; and is unable or unwilling to avail

[1]Interview with Chriz on 10 July 2013. See Appendix 5.1.

L.W. Gitau, *Trauma-Sensitivity and Peacebuilding*, The Anthropocene: Politik—Economics—Society—Science 12, DOI 10.1007/978-3-319-49803-4_5

himself/herself of the protection of that country, or to return there, for fear of persecution (UNHCR 2001: 16).

Possession of citizenship or nationality leads to the enjoyment of services such as education, health care, employment, other basic necessities and overall state protection. People with no citizenship are thus some of the most vulnerable in the world. The UNHCR seeks to provide international protection for refugees who are covered by its Statute and by the 1951 Refugee Convention (UNHCR 2012), hence Chriz's emphasis in the interview excerpt above of the importance of being registered as a refugee and acquiring the ration card. The UNHCR also works to avert statelessness where it is deemed to be at risk. For example, UNHCR was engaged in 'supporting and monitoring effective implementation of nationality laws in the Republic of Sudan and South Sudan' due to the risk of statelessness for a large number of people of South Sudanese origin living in the north after South Sudan's independence in July 2011 (UNHCR 2012). The UNHCR acts as the lead agency in the co-ordination and provision of refugee assistance, and monitors relief programmes which are delivered by its implementing partners consisting of NGOs, the host government, and intergovernmental agencies such as the World Food Programme (WFP) (UNHCR 2012).

Attending to basic human needs after a traumatic experience is crucial to recovery, not just on the physical level, but the psychological level as well. Feeny/Zoellner (2014) underscore this importance, based on their experience

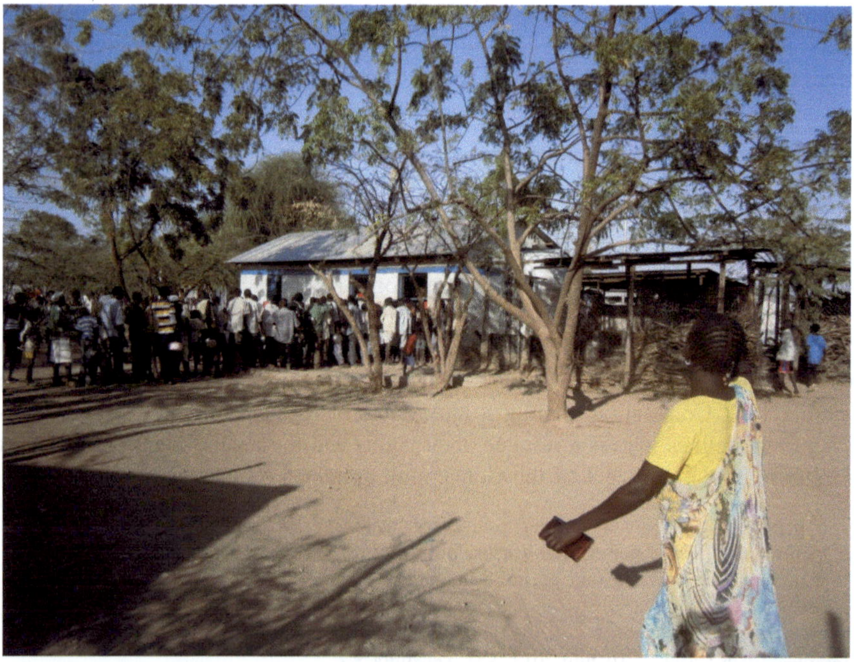

Refugees queue for food at the Kakuma Refugee Camp Reception Centre. *Source* The Author

working on a project in which they were to screen people for mental health difficulties soon after trauma, but found that people kept asking them for housing vouchers, clothing and food assistance. They point out:

> We should not underestimate the psychological power of food, water, sleep, clothing, shelter, and ways to contact family and friends. In the aftermath of natural disasters and in war-torn locations, these basic needs… allow for calming, for a sense of safety, and for predictability to begin to be restored… In the immediate aftermath of trauma, no matter our training, often the best psychological help we can give is delivered in boxes and bottles (Feeny/Zoellner 2014: 326–327).

This was also my experience as a volunteer counsellor in Internally Displaced People's (IDP) camps in Kenya during the 2007–2008 post-election violence. We were there to offer psychological first aid and counselling for the survivors, but increasingly we found that the people were more interested in the basic necessities we could provide, and were most keen to have their names written down on lists that seemed to hold a promise that their needs for housing and other provisions would be met.

The importance survivors place on basic necessities during and in the aftermath of violent conflict makes an examination of the way they are delivered imperative. Is the way the provisions are delivered sensitive enough to the survivors' needs, and does it address the trauma experienced as a result of violence and displacement in any way? Does it weaken or strengthen the refugees? Harrell-Bond (1999) problematizes the idea of the support received by the refugees from UNHCR and its partnering agencies and asks:

> Is it possible that the way refugees are 'helped' is one source of debilitating stress for those who are in a position where they have no alternative but to receive? (Harrell-Bond 1999: 136).

By tracing literature and research with refugees from different countries including Somali refugees in London, Vietnamese refugees in Canada, Bosnian refugees, South Sudanese refugees, and Ugandan refugees among others, and doing a comparative study with Saharawi refugees who manage themselves, Harrell-Bond (1999) concludes that the way aid is given to refugees contributes to their stress. Amongst other things, she raises issue with the tendency to 'depersonalize' refugees, which accompanies assistance programmes, treating refugees as 'homogeneous, undifferentiated masses' and thereby robbing them of human dignity (Harrell-Bond 1999: 140–141). The experience of the loss of status, and having to depend on strangers for basic survival needs, impacts heavily on the self-esteem and dignity of the refugees. Harrell-Bond further takes issue with the contemporary 'repackaging' of refugees as 'helpless, starving masses who depend on agents of compassion to keep them alive' (Harrell-Bond 1999: 147). The repackaging of the refugee thus does not seem to take into consideration the effect it has on the refugee. Harrell-Bond concludes:

> In short, the application of the welfare model, combined with the reality of refugees' initial relative powerlessness in the new environment, tends… to attract and condition the behavior of helpers whose interests are served by pathologizing, medicalizing and labelling the refugee as 'helpless and vulnerable' (Harrell-Bond 1999: 153).

Having thus been rendered 'helpless and vulnerable' by the method in which aid is provided, some refugees have recourse to dramatising their situation and their burdens to the aid workers and other people to draw attention to themselves and receive help. This was the case with Sara, a 30 year old woman from the Nuer community who exhibited epileptic symptoms and demanded to be removed from where she was residing to a safer, more comfortable location, and be treated in a special way. I met and interviewed Sara at the Kakuma Reception Centre where she had run away to from her residence in the camp, claiming that her 'co-wife'[2] was beating her up and that since she was pregnant and unsafe, she needed special attention and care. Sara told me that she had a 'mental' problem, and the interpreter described Sara's epileptic symptoms as 'terrible'. She had come to the Reception Centre a few days previously and the security had tried to chase her away from the gate and she had fallen down. Sara went on to describe her problem to me:

> *Something happened to my head ... even the two of you* [referring to the interpreter and I], *it would be terrible for you to touch me. Because... I'd try to beat someone myself, and if you run away very fast and then maybe there is water there, I'll fall in it, and then ... there is a time I fell down and ... What I need, I don't want to hear some people quarrelling, or people shouting. That causes problems. And I don't, shouldn't be angry too much. Or maybe have lack of food. That's something that causes me this problem also... If we have some people that are shouting, or maybe quarrelling, that problem that I have is awakened...*[3]

In her vulnerable and desperate state, Sara seems to be finding meaning in her 'mental problem' as she calls it, the one condition in which she seems to have control. She talks of what she needs, what she cannot stand, and what triggers her problem. People need to maintain peace and quiet around her, and both anger and hunger are triggers. The condition gives her occasion to oppose the forces or powers that have rendered her vulnerable and helpless.

In his treatise on the social experience of pain, Kleinman (1996) describes a similar scenario in which, Mrs. Mullen, a thirty-year-old married woman from a poor Irish American family, has suffered from severe migraine headaches for over five years, and on close examination of the dynamics surrounding her illness, is seen to be using pain as a form of resistance to the social conditions that force her into her poor, vulnerable state. Kleinman (1996: 140) observes:

> Pushed up against the limits of control and meaning making, poor and oppressed patients may take up whatever is at hand to respond to adversity… Thus, Mrs. Mullen's pain also represents a kind of solution, albeit compromised, to the consequences of dwelling in a world of suffering. … The pain becomes a means of resisting her husband's irresponsibility and her mother's cruel manipulations. Her sense that her world is not her own, that she has no central, secure place in it, is replaced by illness behavior through which Mrs. Mullen, with surprising energy and efficacy, moves to the center of that world and even comes to dominate its flow.

---

[2]The term 'co-wife' is used in polygamous contexts, in this case referring to the other woman with whom Sara shares a husband. In Sara's case, she had three co-wives, two of whom lived back in South Sudan.

[3]Interview with Sara on 4 July 2013. See Appendix 5.1.

Sara, like Mrs. Mullen, is in a sense relegitimizing herself and her dignity as a person in a world that has stripped her of all dignity and sense of control, by dramatising her symptoms and demanding special attention. This calls for sensitivity in the way the basic necessities are provided to the survivors, seeking to respect the survivors' human dignity, and desisting from entrenching feelings of helplessness and powerlessness in the survivors.

5.2 Resilience

A number of participants portrayed other ways of coping with traumatic experiences besides waiting to receive provisions from UNHCR and its partnering agencies. These ways of coping point to the resilience of some of the survivors of the conflict and mass violence. As conceptualized by Hobfoll/de Jong (2014: 70–71), resilience is here understood to mean the ability to withstand negative consequences of traumatic challenges, recover quickly from any symptoms of pathology that may develop, and remain enthusiastic, committed and engaged in important life tasks and produce positive outcomes. Resilience entails a shift of focus from pathology, a pattern of recovery to prior functioning, and identifying and mobilizing resources to cope with the traumatic experiences and thrive (Zoellner/Feeny 2014).

Certain characteristics were evident among those participants who portrayed resilience, as shown in the figure below. The characteristics are interconnected and mutually reinforcing. Each of the characteristics is examined below as expressed by the participants (Fig. 5.1).

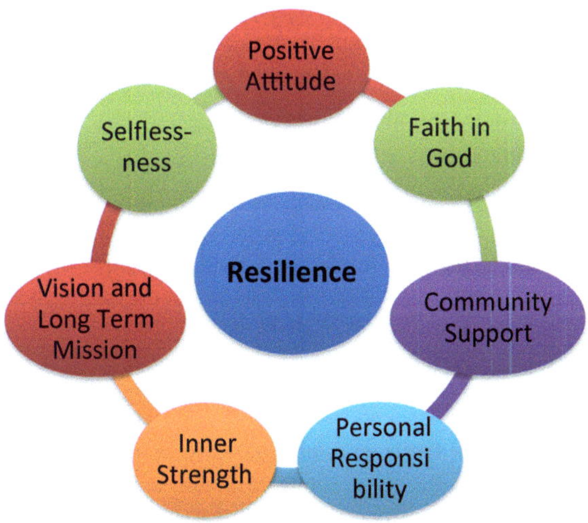
Positive Attitude
Faith in God
Selfless-ness
Resilience
Vision and Long Term Mission
Community Support
Inner Strength
Personal Responsi bility

Fig. 5.1 Other ways of coping. *Source* The author

5.2.1 *Positive Attitude:* 'What Has Happened Has Passed'

One of these ways of coping was the ability to choose one's attitude and focus on the positive. Atem, a 42 year old man from the Dinka community, clearly demonstrates this choice of a positive attitude when his first child is taken away from him during the skirmishes back in South Sudan, but eventually happily reunited with him and his family in the camp. His is a deliberate decision and effort to focus on the positive, as a way of moving on in his life, as he describes:

> *Yes I'm hopeful. On my side I'm hopeful because I tried. I lost all the parents, even my brothers and sisters, and now I'm just staying, and as you can see, my mood never changes. You should see me in my compound, playing with my children. If you have time you come home, I can invite you to see them, the way I interact with them, and the way we just chat. Even when I just get home, they come to me running and say, 'Hey... baba..!' and then I just feel very fresh and then I just talk to them, from the smallest one, to the biggest one... I forget the past. And now I'm starting the new life. Yes.*[4]

This attitude extends to how one relates with others, as described by Fazila:

> *...with me now, when I have peace within me, it means I don't have hatred for somebody, I don't have jealousy may be for something, I'm yeah, I love everyone, and for me really I just like peace so much, I don't know ... I just feel I have peace. Peace of mind, peace of heart. And I just feel if everyone in Sudan could feel the same, then there will be peace.*[5]

An attitude of gratitude, and recognition of what is working in their favour, even if in the very least, is also a major mark of resilience. One of the most striking refugees I interviewed was 29 year old Rachel who had recently arrived from South Sudan after the murder of her husband. She was a naturally joyful, lively, vibrant woman, in stark contrast with most other refugees. She began the interview by singing a song for me, which she described as a peace song:

> *Salamu Salamu, oiyeye [Peace Peace, oiyeye]*
> *Salaam alaykum, aha [the Peace be upon you, aha]*
> *Salamu Salamu, oiyeye [Peace Peace, oiyeye]*
> *Salaam alaykum, aha... [the Peace be upon you, aha...]*
> *It's a peace song, in Sudan. Yeah yeah yeah.*[6]

Jerem and Joy similarly demonstrated this grateful, positive attitude in their circumstances:

> *What has happened, has passed. And since there is still suffering and people being killed in Sudan, we just pray to God to just make peace be in Sudan, so that people will live in peace. Yeah. What has happened is gone, and people have died enough.*[7]

---

[4]Interview with Atem on 2 July 2013. See Appendix 5.1.

[5]Interview with Fazila on 5 July 2013. See Appendix 5.1.

[6]Interview with Rachel on 9 July 2013. See Appendix 5.1.

[7]Interview with Jerem on 13 July 2013. See Appendix 5.1.

OK. Me I think life is not that very bad in the camp. Cos there is no way that you can be totally in a very bad situation without any help. We have a lot of services and structures that can help.[8]

This positive attitude seems crucial in dealing with the aftermath of violent conflict and negotiating the challenges of displacement that the participants face in the camp. Zolli/Healy (2012: 127) describe the innate personality traits of optimism and confidence as some of the most protective assets against life's stressors. Krystal (2004: 68–69) similarly argues:

> … a "healthy" infantile omnipotence is the most important asset for dealing with life's stresses and potential trauma… It is the emotional mainspring of extraordinary reserves. It provides a profound, unshakeable conviction of one's invulnerability…Individuals who have a healthy dose of the adult residuals of infantile narcissism can preserve their optimism in situations of stress and danger. They are able to retain initiative in their thinking, in their planning, or even just in their fantasy. Even when under severe stress, they manage to recognize the chances of improving the dangerous situation at varying degrees of risk.

In the aftermath of traumatic events back in their country of origin and in their circumstances in the camp, these participants are able to make a choice of how to respond, and the choice influences their actions and their relationships.

5.2.2 *Community Support:* 'They Stay with Me Well'

The South Sudanese community highly values living together and sharing whatever they have with one another, and the community members support each other in the midst of difficult circumstances. This is a mark of resilience in the sense that through this support, the survivors are able to withstand the consequences of traumatic events in their lives. Atem, a community leader, aptly expresses the communal way in which the South Sudanese community lives in the camp:

...about the life of the people who are living in the camp, we live together, and even the host community...I invite them also to come to my group. We stay as neighbours and we stay as brothers and sisters. They come, some take water and take food, and we share what we have and then we interact with them.[9]

Zeneb also describes this community spirit when she says:

And there is also something we call help: I help you, also you help others. So, if I get help, now, and have that piece of education that I need, I'll be willing and able to help some others, also. Yeah.[10]

[8]Interview with Joy on 16 July 2013. See Appendix 5.1.

[9]Interview with Atem on 2 July 2013. See Appendix 5.1.

[10]Interview with Zeneb on 3 July 2013. See Appendix 5.1.

Another mark of this communal essence of life amongst the South Sudanese refugees is the willingness, indeed assumed duty of the elders of the community, to give wisdom and guidance to the younger generation whenever it is needed. Paulo, who had lost both parents in the war and had to take care of his younger brother as well as other young children, described how he was advised by the elders about taking responsibility and being an example to the younger ones.

40 year old Grace from the Acholi community described the invaluable support she receives from her group of fellow survivors of HIV/AIDS:

> *That's how I stay. Sometimes I stay, and I find the problems are too many, and I go back to those friends of mine, the ones I counted for you... Those ones will help me. Even them, sometimes if they are facing those issues, they will come, we talk together, and there is peace. For us. …Now these ones sometimes, when we stay together, everyone speaks out their problem, each person their problem, then when we, when everyone has said their problem, then the counsellor, we stay with the counsellor, ...And then some other people, like now those children, they come to visit me, they stay with me, like the way you have come and found us, and we stay together. They stay with me well.*[11]

Community support is especially important for the survivors because of the breakdown in ties resulting from conflict and mass violence back in their country of origin, and they continue to experience in the camp, having lost or been separated from loved ones as well as torn apart from their communities.

In her study of resilience in South Sudanese refugee women, Wanga-Odhiambo (2014) discusses the potency of social ties in dealing with the broken down social fabric and describes how the South Sudanese refugee women in Nairobi formed self-help groups and associations to support one another. One such group, the Sudanese Women's Association in Nairobi (SWAN) was registered in Kenya as a non-profit humanitarian association, and had membership from different cities in Kenya as well as Kakuma refugee camp, camps in Uganda, and overseas (Wanga-Odhiambo 2014: 121). The groups sought to attend to the physical, emotional, psychological, spiritual and cultural needs of the members.

Feeny/Zoellner (2014) emphasize the need to support the meaningful societal ties in order to promote resilience. Community support entails rebuilding trust and the capacity to trust that have been torn away by conflict and violence (Maynard 1999). This is crucial for the restoration of the society to function once again. As Kleber et al. (1995: 304) argues:

> Society provides people with "tools" in relation to the aftermath of traumatic experiences. Norms and values as well as symbols and rituals channel thoughts and emotions and consequently create opportunities for individual ways of adjustment… Cultural belief systems, along with cultural objects and social role expectations, greatly affect psychosocial adjustment in individuals attempting to master severe trauma.

[11]Interview with Grace on 17 July 2013. See Appendix 5.1.

5.2.3 *A Vision and Long-Term Mission:* 'I Have a Passion'

A vision or a long term mission, seemed to be a key ingredient for resilience in some of the participants. A number of the participants, such as Kerieme below, portrayed their long term goal of going back to South Sudan in the future, and helping to bring peace to the nation:

> *In future, my vision. My vision, I just want to complete my study, and then to go back if peace comes, to go back to my motherland and then to work ... then to help my people, to help my people.*[12]

Fazila was particularly ambitious and optimistic of acquiring education and being able to influence the political situation in her country in future for the better:

> *So by getting education, I just think it will help me a lot and it will help not only me but my people also, my family, my people back in Sudan. I'll use it to empower people also...so I'm looking forward to maybe go to university, study, achieve my goals, and my dreams. I go to Sudan, in whatever means I have to work for peace... What I want... I have a burden, I have a passion of people stopping fighting in Sudan, because it is actually... People have shed blood for many many years. I was told when I was just born, people were already fighting. I don't know for what, and I want to know the reasons why these people really fighting, and they are just one nation. So I want to stop war, by any means.*[13]

Nafy[14] was aiming to be a journalist in South Sudan after completing her education, and saw herself involved in such missions as bringing the different South Sudanese tribal communities together through such activities as sports.

The larger vision of not only improving life in the camp, and one's personal life at that, propels this particular group of people beyond the immobilization, powerlessness and despair, symptoms of trauma expressed by some participants, as described in Chap. 5. This was further expressed by Riek and by Jean Paul, a 23 year old man from the Nuer community.

> *I have long term mission. That's why I'm still unmarried...I have more capacity in leadership management. Because I have been trained by the UN over and over ... On how to manage the community.... and how to manage people ... give them counsel, and so on.*[15]

> *As for me, as for me, yes I can say, at long last, yes I can go back for the purpose of saying let me go, and tell people this is not the right way, but this is the way to go.... My hope, if I will grow up as now I'm growing to be an elder, or to be a big person, is to change my country to be a good country.... It is to change my people to be a good people. It is to change the society to know how they can live, and how they can stay with others.*[16]

---

[12]Interview with Kerieme on 4 July 2013. See Appendix 5.1.

[13]Interview with Fazila on 5 July 2013. See Appendix 5.1.

[14]Interview with Nafy on 5 July 2013. See Appendix 5.1.

[15]Interview with Riek on 11 July 2013. See Appendix 5.1.

[16]Interview with Jean Paul on 15 July 2013. See Appendix 5.1.

They have a goal they are living for, and this helps them to overcome the paralyzing power of unpredictability and lack of control that threatens their lives as refugees (Krystal 2004).

5.2.4 *Selflessness:* 'My Heart Is for Everyone'

A key attribute of these refugees demonstrating resilience is a focus beyond the self, and a remarkable leadership quality. Many of them described how they had poured their lives into causes beyond themselves, and this seemed to enable them to thrive despite their dire circumstances. Abit, a 35 year old man from the Dinka community, described his mission of preaching peace to the rest of the community, for instance:

> *Like now, I'm working as a volunteer. But I also like to tell the people how the work is going, and how the peace is going… to tell the people how to stay in peace. That is what I'm doing… Like if you get a place where there are some people near to fight you go and tell them 'hey, hey, hey, wait for me', and you also to tell them how the peace is going.*[17]

Paulo, Matida (a 28 year old woman from the Nuba community), and Jean Paul are examples of youth who found themselves entrusted or in charge of a number of young children whose parents' whereabouts no one knew. In giving of themselves to help out, their strength is drawn and grows:

> *But when I came here you know I have to do something for the children that were left behind. Like when I come, cos since I'm living with the old woman, I have also to cook for those children.*[18]

> *I have three, and my sister's sons three also, and another one, they are seven…. I'm just alone, and these kids they are very small, I'll not be able to leave them just alone like that, because no one else can help them, that's what makes me to struggle with them.*[19]

Jean Paul gave up going on with secondary education when his long lost younger brother joined him in the camp, so that he could give the younger brother an opportunity to go to school as well. When his younger brother joined him in the camp, however, he came accompanied by five other children, unaccompanied minors, whom Jean Paul takes care of as well, as 'the fostering family head' as he put it.[20]

Fazila, as she waits to join university, gives of her time to train children in primary school on peace.[21] Rachel can speak seven different South Sudanese languages, and gives her time to interpret for the camp officials when they speak to the refugees in different forums.[22]

---

[17]Interview with Abit on 2 July 2013. See Appendix 5.1.

[18]Interview with Paulo on 11 July 2013. See Appendix 5.1.

[19]Interview with Matida on 4 July 2013. See Appendix 5.1.

[20]Interview with Jean Paul on 15 July 2013. See Appendix 5.1.

[21]Interview with Fazila on 5 July 2013. See Appendix 5.1.

[22]Interview with Rachel on 9 July 2013. See Appendix 5.1.

Riek, a young man who suffered greatly back home when he lost both parents and his wife-to-be and baby during delivery, is now a leader of his community in the camp and spends most of his time deliberating on intra and intertribal peacebuilding issues in the camp. He described his focused leadership strategies and his then current involvement in a conflict between his community, Nuer, and the Murle community over an alleged abduction of a child by the latter from the Nuer community. Riek described his involvement in peacebuilding:

> *As a leader, I'm also a counsellor. People bring cases to me all the time. Currently, I'm dealing with the issue of the clashes between the Nuer and the Murle, in which 7 people were killed, 5 Murle, and 2 Nuer. As a leader, I was suspected of inciting my people, but I proved to the authorities my innocence, and told them I work as a peacemaker in my community, and if I was a violent person I could not hold these positions. Together with other stakeholders, we are working to reunite the two communities. I've been very busy holding meetings with my people and other joint meetings with all stakeholders, to try to reconcile the two communities.*[23]

Jerem, a pastor of the Nuba community in the camp talks of his concern for the youth and the possibility of establishing a library in the church to improve the welfare of the young people:

> *If there could be an establishment of a library, that could be of help to people because they could be staying around here and at least studying about the word of God...I feel there is nothing that can help me only. My heart is for everyone and I think everyone could be assisted, not me alone.*[24]

Krystal (2004), in discussing how some of the Holocaust survivors coped through atrocious experiences, underscores the power of love, and describes how the capacity for loving and serving others provided a means of preserving hope and faith, maintaining a sense of one's own humanity, and protecting oneself from withdrawal and surrender. Krystal (2004: 77) concludes:

> Most of all there is the clear indication that one's resilience is proportional to the capacity to mobilize one's love powers. Love outraged is experienced as anger or hate. Love rendered helpless manifest itself as shame. However, love represents the survivor's self-reintegrating and self-healing powers.

Kaminer/Eagle (2010: 73) note that traumatic experiences can cause survivors to develop an increased compassion and empathy for others, as 'their personal experience of trauma allows for a richer emotional insight into the pain and distress of other people'. This leads to involvement in self-giving activities that result in deeper feelings of connection to other people, which facilitates recovery from trauma (Herman 1997).

---

[23]Interview with Riek on 11 July 2013. See Appendix 5.1.

[24]Interview with Jerem on 13 July 2013. See Appendix 5.1.

5.2.5 *Faith in God:* 'Only Just Tell God'

The South Sudanese refugee community in Kakuma is highly religious. In a significant way, their faith, acts as a means of coping amidst the difficult situation both in their country and in the camp. There seems to be an assumed question, 'How else would you, or anyone, make sense of any of the things that have happened, and still live on?' which their faith answers. Like Fazila, most of the refugees believe every step of their journey is through God's intervention:

> *I believe it is the mercies of God, maybe. Yeah, I just believe every step I take it is God who is leading me. In order to go and establish peace.*[25]

Most clusters of homesteads (blocks) in the South Sudanese community in the camp have a structure made up of a low mud hedge and long mud benches, which the refugees described as a place of worship. Their belief in God is the source of hope, and the only cord they can hold on to in order to be saved from annihilation, as it were. Rachel said of her belief in God:

> *Only just tell God, I know God helps me… if I feel badly and I cry, if I cry say at night, tomorrow I wake up happy… I know God is with me… My God is great, and is doing something big in my life.*[26]

These individuals' faith enables them to negotiate their pain and trauma and make meaning of it, experience healing, and extend help to others. As Puljek-Shank/Puljek-Shank (2008: 180) found out in their work on trauma healing and peacebuilding in South Eastern Europe, this experience that transforms pain and suffering into a source of strength is both deeply spiritual and effective in helping people cope with the consequences of traumatic events. Krystal (2004: 78) also found faith to be a strong determinant of resilience for Holocaust survivors:

> An inner resource of enormous power was the ability to maintain some sense of continuing identification with something transcendental that would endure: God… some "higher power.

5.2.6 *Taking Personal Initiative and Agency:* 'Even Little by Little It Helps'

Stories of the refugees' personal initiatives in the face of difficult circumstances are particularly poignant. Kakuma Refugee Camp is situated in a very remote and arid part of Kenya, and economically resourceful projects are an uphill task even in normal circumstances. Yet a number of refugees make a remarkable attempt at improving their circumstances by trying out different enterprises.

[25]Interview with Fazila on 5 July 2013. See Appendix 5.1.

[26]Interview with Rachel on 9 July 2013. See Appendix 5.1.

Zeneb's mother had, after her husband had gone back to South Sudan and been killed, started a small business of selling vegetables in the market, and saved enough money to send her daughter (Zeneb) to a good school in Nairobi.[27]

Jerem supplements his family's upkeep by making traditional wooden beds for sale in the camp.[28] Dabor fled from South Sudan after her husband was killed in the war, as she was afraid that her children would be recruited as child soldiers. While in the camp, she had got married again, and her second husband had also died in the war. With five children to fend for, she tried what she could, as she described:

> *So we just try, if I get a little flour, I make 'mandazi' [doughnuts], and sell outside. Whatever little I get, it helps me get some soap, onion, and so on.*[29]

Grace, who has HIV/AIDS and is currently supporting nine children of her deceased brother, and one of her own, tries to make ends meet and supplement their diet through a food business that she started. She said:

> *Just recently I started this [business], people come and eat and I get some money... Yeah, I cook this ... porridge and mandazi [doughnuts]. So I get a little money, sometimes I buy vegetables. Together with the ration food they give us ... Even little by little it helps... I sometimes just buy, 'sukuma' [kale]... then we stay.*[30]

An overarching theme in the resilient group of refugees is a sense of agency. Agency, as defined by Goddard (2000: 27), refers to 'the capacity of individuals or groups to embark on processes of autonomous self-realization.' Sen (1999) underscores the importance of recognising, understanding and enhancing the agency of the people in need of assistance and argues:

> Understanding the agency role is thus central to recognizing people as responsible persons: not only are we well or ill, but also we act or refuse to act, and can choose to act one way rather than another. And thus we – women and men – must take responsibility for doing things or not doing them. It makes a difference, and we have to take note of that difference. This elementary acknowledgement, though simple enough in principle, can be exacting in its implications, both for social analysis and for practical reason and action (Sen 1999: 190).

For the South Sudanese survivors in the camp, agency entails a sense of being able to influence and direct their own lives, even if in the smallest sense of the word, in the midst of devastating conditions. This is in stark contrast to the resignation and powerlessness expressed by some participants, as described in Chap. 5. Rachel for instance denotes this ability to take matters in her own hands in her adamant refusal to be taken advantage of through wife-inheritance by her brother-in-law, after her husband died in the war:

> *Yes I refused and said let me just take care of these five children. I don't want. He chased me away from home. He said you go, if you want to leave. He insulted me badly... I was even about to go crazy... Every time I went to try and find a job, he didn't care about me.*

[27]Interview with Zeneb on 3 July 2013. See Appendix 5.1.

[28]Interview with Jerem on 13 July 2013. See Appendix 5.1.

[29]Interview with Dabor on 16 July 2013. See Appendix 5.1.

[30]Interview with Grace on 17 July 2013. See Appendix 5.1.

He was insulting me, calling me Malaya (prostitute) because I refused. He treated me badly too much. So I said let me go to the refugee scheme, they can be able to help me. Even now he wants to come to take the three children from me … The other two children, my father has them… I took them to school… because they were both in school the time my husband died and they said they will not leave the school because of the death of my husband…[31]

Chriz portrayed this agency through a rare interest in my work as a researcher, and what it would achieve towards conflict resolution and alleviating the people's suffering in South Sudan and other places. He expressed his anxiety about the results of my research. He asked me:

Ok. What is your… what do you want to do about these conflicts in the countries where people are suffering? Is there anything you'd like to make to stop wars and conflicts?,,, Yeah, I'm so anxious about the result of it.[32]

Suleyman made the decision and took the initiative to flee to the camp when he got the opportunity, after assessing the situation back home and seeing nothing positive coming out of it. This is in contrast with other refugees who fled for safety, having no option, and not pausing to consider their circumstances:

So when I saw life is bad, I got a chance of coming here, so I decided on my own, then I came. … Yeah because there was nothing at all. From the beginning, up to the end, there's nothing good, that I've seen in my life. And for all the entire people… Yeah, that's why, when I got a chance I came. I flew to one of the NGOs, that is NCA: Norwegian Church Aid. They helped me to fly from there to South Sudan, then from there I used the roads to reach Kenya.[33]

Patrick had taken the initiative to move his family out of danger from his home to Juba, before eventually moving them to the camp.

Yeah. Good thing this time now, during that attack of last year I sent my wife and little children to Juba, in the town. I was the only one person there with the rest of the family. They are now okay. (hesitantly) looking okay… They are here now. Some of them I've tried to send them to the school now.[34]

Joy talks of having 'developed courage' through her stay in the camp, and hence trying out ways of improving her circumstances:

I developed courage that I can do like any other person. Also whenever I have problem, I felt it's only what you can plan to make you cope with the situation. It's not that UNHCR or any other agencies are there to support you. They can support you, but not always.[35]

One of Joy's personal initiatives is starting a 'merry-go-round'[36] self-help group amongst her colleagues, which has gone a long way in meeting urgent personal financial needs and supplementing their own and their families' diet.

---

[31]Interview with Rachel on 9 July 2013. See Appendix 5.1.

[32]Interview with Chriz on 10 July 2013. See Appendix 5.1.

[33]Interview with Suleyman on 10 July 2013. See Appendix 5.1.

[34]Interview with Patrick on 15 and 16 July 2013. See Appendix 5.1.

[35]Interview with Joy on 16 July 2013. See Appendix 5.1.

[36]A 'merry-go-round' as used here refers essentially to a group of people, mostly women, who contribute funds on a monthly basis and distribute them on a rotational basis to members of the

The concept of agency is crucial to resilience. The individual or group is an active agent in the adaptation process, makes deliberate effort and takes certain choices in response to the adversity. In their analytical disaggregation of agency, Emirbayer/Mische (1998: 971–972) posit three constitutive elements of agency that make this process of adaptation possible, namely *iteration, projectivity* and *practical evaluation. Iteration* refers to the ability of individuals or groups to select past patterns of thought and action and incorporate them into the present situation, and in effect enable a sense of continuity and order in the universe, even in difficult situations. *Projectivity* refers to the ability of individuals or groups to imagine future possibilities and think of creative ways of confronting present fears and fulfilling their hopes and desires for the future. *Practical evaluation* refers to the capacity of individuals and groups 'to make practical and normative judgments among alternative possible trajectories of action, in response to the emerging demands, dilemmas, and ambiguities' (Emirbayer/Mische 1998: 971).

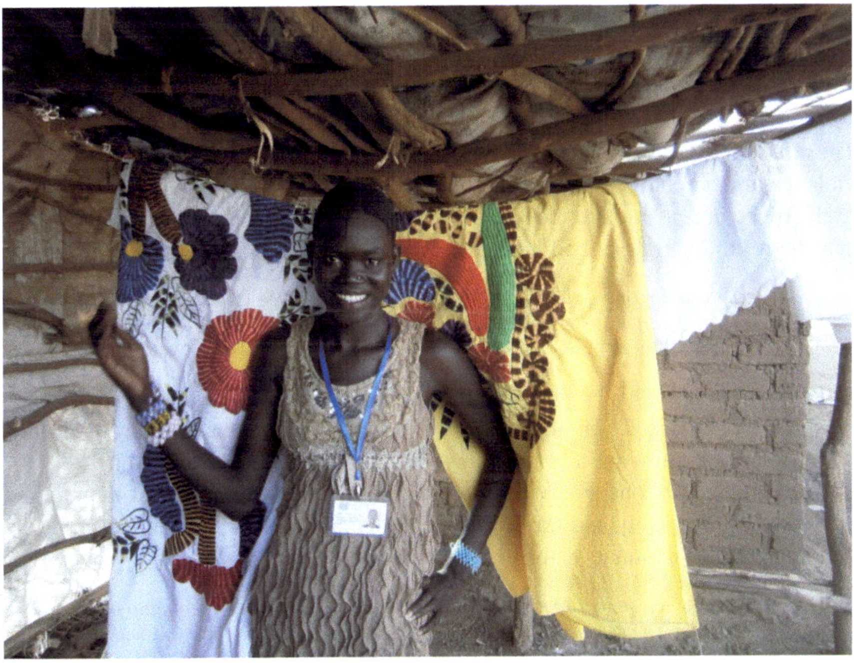

A refugee at Kakuma poses with some samples of her embroidery work. *Source* The Author. Photo used with permission from Teresa Achol

(Footnote 36 continued)

group. The concept of a merry-go-round has been used widely by women's self-help groups in Kenya (Jussi et al. 2009).

Restoring people's capacity to make choices in their lives is one key way of fostering resilience to adversity. Resilient people are said to have an 'internal locus of control'—a sense of being able to affect their own destiny (Richters 2010). This renders them more capable of effectively participating in poverty reduction programmes. Individual resilience thus provides a key to addressing the overlapping causes and effects of conflict and poverty in order to promote peacebuilding and development after mass violence (Lambourne/Gitau 2013). Chandler argues for a 'bottom-up' understanding of human security, in which the emphasis is no longer upon the intervening actors, but on empowering the people in need of assistance (Chandler 2012: 223). In positing the resilience debate against the human security interventionist paradigm, Chandler (2012: 216), in accord with Sen's (1999) ideas on agency, argues that a resilience paradigm 'puts agency of those most in need of assistance at the centre, stressing a programme of empowerment and capacity-building'. This shifts the focus from state-based to society-based understanding of security practices, which include the interventions survivors of conflict and mass violence receive. Chandler sees this as a necessity, not an option, since the premise of security in the first place is the inability of those being secured to secure themselves, hence the need to enhance their agency.

5.2.7 *Inner Strength:* 'We Tried to Manage'

The refugees from South Sudan had struggled against many odds to survive the mass violence in their country and clearly, being able to get to Kakuma Refugee Camp in itself and be in a position to receive the UNHCR provisions in the camp, was a great achievement. Atem described how he managed to get to Kakuma and get help:

> *And then I started running away, and then we tried to manage ... that's when I came to Kakuma. Then I started living here in Kakuma.... I tried to manage ... when I came here life was become difficult to me, and I tried to manage.*[37]

Riek had to leave his home as a result of insecurity, when he learnt he was being pursued. When I asked him how he had coped, he said that he had basically decided to concentrate on finding a practical way of getting out of the situation.[38]

The camp conditions are evidently not ideal but a good number of the refugees learn to cope creatively and thrive despite the circumstances. Miriam describes her determination to continue with life in the camp:

> *I was just struggling, so that I finish my school and then I see what I'm going to do, but life it is not easy. Sometimes you may find the food is not enough, and then you will stay with hunger three or four days, if you don't have anybody who has a job, until you wait for the ration to come and then you go and collect your food.*[39]

---

[37]Interview with Atem on 2 July 2013. See Appendix 5.1.

[38]Interview with Riek on 11 July 2013. See Appendix 5.1.

[39]Interview with Joy on 16 July 2013. See Appendix 5.1.

Jean Paul described how he had, at a young age, suddenly become a 'foster parent' to six other children who had arrived in the camp accompanying his younger brother. Asked how he coped, he said:

> *It is to understand. You understand them and they understand you… Whatever idea you have, you give them. Then they understand about life. They understand your idea, you accept what they are saying, then you advise them how they should go to school, and which time they are supposed to be at home, and how they should prepare some lunch and supper, that's the idea.*[40]

The knack for survival even amidst difficult situations is repeatedly portrayed amongst the refugees. Joy for example is a mother of two, about to give birth to her third child. She describes how she takes care of her children on her own as her husband is estranged. She presents a very buoyant personality in her manner. Grace, who contracted HIV/AIDS after being raped by a soldier back in South Sudan and being forced to marry him, has given birth 14 times and only one child has survived so far. She has subsequently lost other relatives including a brother and his wife, and been left to care for ten children. Amidst all she has gone through, Grace remains jovial, hopeful and good-humoured.

These are the kind of people whom Krystal (2004: 73) describes as having 'hidden vestigial optimism [which] permitted some limited alertness and initiative, even inventiveness.'

Kaminer/Eagle (2010) discuss how experiencing trauma can lead to positive changes in perceptions of the self. Survivors of a traumatic experience may find deep inner reserves of strength which were not apparent before the traumatic experience, and may be able to draw from these reserves to cope with the trauma, and help others. In discussing their work on trauma healing and peacebuilding in South Eastern Europe, Puljek-Shank/Puljek-Shank (2008: 180) refer to this great potential that exists in the pain of trauma for transformation to something positive, and explain how some of the people they have worked with have come to use their trauma as a source of strength and compassion for others. The South Sudanese participants discussed in this section manifested this potential in the way they managed to function positively in their circumstances, and even reach out to others.

5.3 Community Resilience

To the extent that life for the South Sudanese refugees is community-oriented, the concept of community resilience would apply to the case of the participants of this research. The concept of collective trauma as described in Chap. 3, meaning that the impact of mass violence is experienced in relationships in families and the community at large, is one aspect of the community-oriented ways that the South Sudanese refugees experience life. If the experience of trauma is a community concern, then conceptualizing coping with trauma from a community perspective is

[40]Interview with Jean Paul on 15 July 2013. See Appendix 5.1.

of value. The concept of community resilience thus becomes significant in this research. Saul (2014: 8) defines community resilience as:

> A community's capacity, hope and faith to withstand major trauma and loss, overcome adversity, and to prevail, usually with increased resources, competence and connectedness.

Norris et al. (2008: 127) define community resilience as 'a process linking a network of adaptive capacities (resources with dynamic attributes) to adaptation after a disturbance or adversity'. Norris et al. acknowledge the complex interconnectedness of communities to their natural, social and economic environments.

The concept of community resilience extends and develops the idea that a focus on symptoms and effects of trauma on individuals is limited, and embraces the importance of the social context in terms of the social, and cultural, realities which structure the way violence occurs and how people recover (Bracken et al. 1995). Social reality refers to such things as family circumstances, social networks and economic position, and cultural realities refer to such things as language, religion, beliefs, values and concept of self and community.

The idea of identifying, consolidating and mobilizing different resources in order to cope with traumatic experiences resonates with the concept of community resilience (Saul 2014). These resources include the social, political, cultural, religious, and environmental resources. Pickren (2014: 19) points to the immense resource that refugees have in terms of cultural ways in which they engage with the world, and how these ways can be adopted and adapted in their new environments to enable coping.

An application of the Conservation of Resources (COR) theory (Hobfoll/de Jong 2014) can be used to explain the resilience of the South Sudanese participants discussed. This theory holds that 'individuals have a primary motivation to build, maintain, and protect the resources necessary to protect the self, the family, and the tribe' (Hobfoll/de Jong 2014: 73). The theory operates on three principles discussed below (Hobfoll/de Jong 2014: 73–75).

The first principle is that resource loss is disproportionately more powerful than resource gain. In the case of South Sudanese refugees, this is seen to be true when one considers the intensity and amount of destruction of physical, social, cultural and spiritual resources that has accompanied the violence in South Sudan, and how difficult and time-consuming it is to restore these resources, if it is possible at all.

The second principle is that people must invest resources in order to protect against resource loss, recover from losses, and gain resources. In the case of the South Sudanese refugees, this may appear retrospective because the traumatic events have already taken place, but looking at the participants who were found to be resilient, it is evident that they had invested resources that they are now able to draw from in order to negotiate the traumatic experiences, and help others as well.

The third principle states that although resource loss is more powerful than resource gain, the salience of gain increases under situations of resource loss. The state of loss seems to have the ability to stir wells of strength and capacity to transform circumstances for the better, as seen in the participants discussed, for whom even the smallest enterprises can be seen as making a difference in their ability to cope.

Some of the participants in the research, cited in this chapter, draw from inner strength to cope with the traumatic events, and are motivated to serve others and make the best of the situation, rather than succumb to circumstances and stay immobilized. This last principle points to the potential for post-traumatic growth, or what Linley/Joseph (2004: 11) refer to as 'adversarial growth'. Post-traumatic growth or adversarial growth refers to the positive changes that may arise in the process of struggling through the traumatic experience, that motivate the survivors to higher levels of functioning than those that existed before the event.

Saul (2014) also sees the COR theory as applicable in the case of collective trauma. He argues:

> Massive trauma often involves a serious loss of resources… stress occurs when people lose their resources, when they are threatened with resource loss or are unable to develop or enhance resources despite significant effort. Following major traumatic events, those with fewer resources are more deeply impacted and may fall into rapid and turbulent loss cycles in which the loss of one or more resources triggers further losses. Such downward loss spirals, which are extremely difficult to reverse, may lead to anxiety, depression, and loneliness, as well as reduced social involvement, diminished interest in life, feelings of social detachment and a sense of alienation. In order for communities to recover, these vicious loss cycles have to be interrupted and resource gain cycles reintroduced (Saul 2014: 5–6).

In order to reintroduce cycles of resource gain and help a community to recover, the Community Resilience Model (CRM) proposed by Miller-Karas (2015) may offer insight into the process. The CRM is a culturally contextualized model to help communities access their strengths and capacities for healing and recovery. It is based on the concept of 'neuroplasticity', a discovery in the expanding field of neuroscience that acknowledges that the brain is malleable—it can change.

> If the brain can change, then so can our beliefs, feelings, and associated sensations. Specifically, new pathways or connections between neurons can be created within the brain and body. The creation of new neuronal pathways can result in greater resilience (Miller-Karas 2015: 7).

The model is geared towards making interventions for survivors of traumatic experiences 'resilience-informed'. It serves to normalize and de-stigmatize the reactions to traumatic events. Within this model, people learn skills to assist them to get to their 'resilient zone', which represents 'the natural rhythm or flow within the nervous system… where we have a greater capacity for balanced thinking and feeling. We can create the best solutions for our own lives, our families, and our wider community' (Miller-Karas 2015: 33).

The concept of community resilience is thus seen to be relevant and appropriate in the case of South Sudanese survivors in the camp, in helping them withstand the consequences of the traumatic events they have faced, recover, and be committed and engaged in productive activities.

5.4 Conclusion

Provision of basic necessities to the refugees is crucial to their recovery, not only on the physical level, but on the psychological level as well. This underscores the importance of sensitivity to the way these basic necessities are provided. Does it entrench feelings of helplessness in the refugees, or empower and encourage them to cope and thrive in the midst of difficult circumstances?

The concept of resilience as it emerged from the interviews is portrayed in particular characteristics portrayed by some participants, namely a positive attitude, community support, a long term vision and mission, selflessness, faith in God, taking personal initiative and agency, and inner strength. These characteristics, in their interconnectedness and mutually reinforcing nature, are seen to help the participants withstand the consequences of their traumatic experiences and engage in positive and productive activities.

Finally, a focus on the concept of community resilience as a culture- and trauma-sensitive model of recovery is seen to be relevant for South Sudanese survivors in the camp, in helping shift the focus from debilitating circumstances to more positive outcomes, and identify and mobilize resources to cope with traumatic experiences, and even thrive.

Trauma-sensitive interventions that are culturally sensitive and cognizant of the complex and nuanced ways in which people experience conflict, violence and recovery, and at the same time recognize and promote the capacity of the survivors to recover, are seen to assist in recovery and prevention of recurring hatred and violence (Keane 2003; Vasilevska 2014), and as will be seen in the next chapter, to facilitate peacebuilding.

Appendix 5.1

Pseudonym	M/F	Ethnic group	Age	Duration of stay in the camp	Brief details	Date of interview
Grace	F	Acholi	40	14 years	Father and brother tortured and killed on being suspected to be traitors. Raped and forced into marriage by a soldier. Has given birth 14 times and only one child has survived. Also taking care of 10 of her deceased brothers' children. Was diagnosed HIV positive in the camp and resettlement process stalled. Cooks food for sale to supplement the ration in the camp	17th July 2013
Patrick	M	Murle	40	5 months	People from the Nuer Community attacked his village and killed many people, his wife and children ran to the bush where his wife delivered their last child. SPLA soldiers attacked his village, many people were killed and he	15th and 16th July 2013

(continued)

(continued)

Pseudonym	M/F	Ethnic group	Age	Duration of stay in the camp	Brief details	Date of interview
					sustained injuries. Worked as a Livestock officer. In the Reconciliation committee between the Murle and the Nuer in the camp	
Joy	F	Acholi	32	12 years	Fled civil war in South Sudan and came to camp with cousin. Mother joined her in 2003. Was unable to complete secondary education in the camp. Case worker with LWF Peacebuilding unit. Has two children and is expecting a third in a month's time. Separated from her husband	16th July 2013
Suleyman	M	Nuba	27	4 years	Fled discrimination in South Kordofan and joined his brother in the camp. Gave a brief history of the different civil wars and peace attempts between the South and the North. Has received counselling services and training from JRS	10th July 2013
Dabor	F	Didinga	46	20 years	Escaped war between the North and the South. Parents and husband died in the war. Feared her children would be recruited as child soldiers and fled. Remarried in Kakuma, got two other children and second husband also died in the war when he went back to fight. Was working as a midwife in Kakuma hospital but lost her job in 1999. Cooks doughnuts to sell in the camp	16th July 2013
Kerieme	M	Nuba	20	1 month	At the Reception Centre waiting to be settled in the Camp. Came all alone to Kakuma from Yida IDP camp and does not know where other family members are	4th July
Fazila	F	Nuba	21	14 years	Family escaped due to the war between South Sudan and Arabs in 1999. Came to the camp with	5th July 2013

(continued)

(continued)

Pseudonym	M/F	Ethnic group	Age	Duration of stay in the camp	Brief details	Date of interview
					step-mother and two siblings. Father an SPLA. Mother joined them in the camp in 2012. Has won scholarship and is preparing to go to University in Canada in August	
Zeneb	F	Dinka	20	20 years	Born in the camp. Father went back to South Sudan in 1996 and was short dead. Moved to Nairobi with mother in 2003 to attend school. Mother died in 2010 as a result of wounds sustained in the post-election violence in Kenya in 2008. Working as an incentive case worker with Peacebuilding unit of LWF	3rd July 2013
Riek	M	Nuer	27	8 years	Escaped due to insecurity after his parents, fiancée and unborn child died. Has taken advantage of different education opportunities in the camp. Works as a community leader. Involved in reconciliation efforts between the Nuer and the Murle tribes in the camp	8th July 2013
Chriz	M	Nuba	23	7 years	Fled insecurity in South Kordofan. Left family members there. Came to the camp to pursue an education. Completed high school in 2011 and is teaching at Kakuma secondary school	10th July 2013
Sara	F	Nuer	30	1 year	Was married as a fourth wife back in South Sudan. Living with one of the co-wives in the camp. Had run to the Reception Centre seeking shelter as a result of mistreatment from co-wife. Has one child and is pregnant. Is epileptic	4th July 2013
Atem	M	Dinka	42	21 years	Community leader. Married, with four children. Had gone back to South Sudan in 1999 to participate in the war and came	2nd July 2013

(continued)

(continued)

Pseudonym	M/F	Ethnic group	Age	Duration of stay in the camp	Brief details	Date of interview
					back to the camp in 2005. Incentive worker with IRC. Was among 'The Lost Boys'	
Jerem	M	Nuba	50	8 years	Pastor of Nuban Community Church. Father died when he was seven days old. Disowned by family at 17 due to converting from Islam to Christianity. Fled from the Arabs in Sudan. Makes traditional beds for sale in the camp to raise some money	13th July 2013
Nafy	M	Dinka	19	19 years	Born in Kakuma. Family escaped war between the South and the North. Father was killed, mother was married (inherited) by father's brother. Has just completed secondary education in Nakuru, Kenya, through sponsorship. Wants to train to be a journalist	5th July 2013
Paulo	M	Dinka	19	10 years	Went back to South Sudan in 2007 and came back to the camp in 2010. No parents. Living with and taking care of little brother and sister and an old relative	3rd July 2013
Jean Paul	M	Nuer	23	10 years	Fled South Sudan when unknown people attacked his village to raid cattle and every one dispersed. He was shot in the leg. Eventually learnt his parents were killed when he was reunited with his brother in 2012. Also taking care of five other children who came along with his younger brother. Does not know the whereabouts of seven of his siblings. Working in the Reconciliation committee for the Murle and the Nuer tribes in the camp	15th July 2013
Matida	F	Nuba	28	1 month	Escaped the bombing in South Kordofan. Lost three family members. Came to the camp with three of her children, three	4th July 2013

(continued)

(continued)

Pseudonym	M/F	Ethnic group	Age	Duration of stay in the camp	Brief details	Date of interview
					of her sister's children, and one of her brother's children. Does not know where her husband is	
Abit	M	Dinka	35	21 years	Working as a volunteer in peacebuilding in the camp. Was sponsored by someone in Texas USA to go back to school from 2003 to 2006. Was among 'The Lost Boys'	2nd July

References

Bracken, P.J., Giller, J.E. & Summerfield, D. (1995). 'Psychological Responses to War and Atrocity: The Limitations of Current Concepts'. In *Social Science & Medicine*, Vol. 40, No. 8, pp. 1073–1082.

Chandler, D. (2012). 'Resilience and Human Security: The Post-interventionist Paradigm'. In *Security Dialogue*, Vol. 43, No. 3, pp. 213–229.

Emirbayer, M. & Mische, A. (1998). 'What is agency?' In *American Journal of Sociology,* Vol. 103, No. 4, pp. 962–1023.

Feeny, N.C. & Zoellner, L.A. (2014). 'Conclusion: Risk and Resilience Following Trauma Exposure'. In Zoellner, L.A. & Feeny, N.C. (Eds.) *Facilitating Resilience and Recovery Following Trauma.* New York: The Guilford Press, pp. 325–334.

Goddard, A.V. (2000). 'Introduction'. In Goddard, A.V. (Ed.) *Gender, Agency and Change: Anthropological Perspectives.* London: Routledge, pp. 1–31.

Harrell-Bond, B. (1999). 'The Experience of Refugees as Recipients of Aid'. In Ager, A. (Ed.) *Refugees: Perspectives on the Experience of Forced Migration.* London: Continuum, pp. 136–168.

Herman, J. (1997). *Trauma and Recovery.* New York: Basic Books.

Hobfoll, S.E. & De Jong, J.T.V.M. (2014). 'Sociocultural and Ecological Views of Trauma'. In Zoellner, L.A. & Feeny, N.C. (Eds.) *Facilitating Resilience and Recovery Following Trauma,* New York: The Guilford Press, pp. 69–90.

Kaminer, D. & Eagle, G. (2010). *Traumatic Stress in South Africa.* Johannesburg: Wits University Press.

Keane, T.M. (2003). 'A Call to Action: Responding to Social and Humanitarian Crises'. In Green, B.L., Friedman, M.J., de Jong, J.T.V.M., Solomon, S.D., Keane, T.M., Fairbank, J.A., Donelan, B. & Frey-Wouters, E. (Eds.) *Trauma Interventions in War and Peace: Prevention, Practice and Policy.* New York: Kluwer Academic/Plenum Publishers, pp. 351–362.

Kleber, R.J., Figley, C.R. & Gersons, B.P.R. (1995). 'Introduction'. In Kleber, R.J., Figley, C.R. & Gersons (Eds.) *Beyond Trauma: Cultural and Societal Dynamics.* New York: Plenum Press, pp. 1–11.

Kleinman, A. (1996). *Writing at the Margin: Discourse between Anthropology and Medicine.* Berkeley: University of California Press, pp. 121–146.

Krystal, H. (2004). 'Resilience: Accommodation and Recovery'. In Knafo, D. (Ed.) *Living With Terror, Working With Trauma: A Clinician's Handbook*. Lanham: Jason Aronson, pp. 67–82.

Lambourne, W. & Gitau, L. (2013). 'Psychosocial Interventions, Peacebuilding and Development in Rwanda', *Journal of Peacebuilding and Development*. Vol. 8, No. 3, pp. 23–36.

Linley, P.A. & Joseph, S. (2004). 'Positive Change Following Trauma and Adversity: A Review'. *Journal of Traumatic Stress*, Vol. 17, No. 1, pp. 11–21.

Maynard, A.K. (1999). *Healing Communities in Conflict: International Assistance in Complex Emergencies*. New York: Columbia University Press.

Miller-Karas, E. (2015). *Building Resilience to Trauma: The Trauma and Community Resiliency Models*. New York: Routledge.

Norris, F.H., Stevens, S.P., Pfefferbaum, B., Wyche, K.F. & Pfefferbaum, R.L. (2008). 'Community Resilience as a Metaphor, Theory, Set of Capacities, and Strategy for Disaster Readiness'. *Community Psychology*, Vol. 41, pp. 127–150.

Pickren, W.E. (2014). 'What is Resilience and How Does it Relate to the Refugee Experience? Historical and Theoretical Perspectives'. In Simich, L. & Andermann, L. (Eds.) *Refuge and Resilience: International Perspectives on Migration*. New York: Springer, pp. 7–26.

Puljek-Shank, A. & Puljek-Shank, R. (2008). 'The Contribution of Trauma Healing to Peacebuilding in South East Europe'. In Hart, B. (Ed.) *Peacebuilding in Traumatized Societies*. New York: University Press of America, pp. 155–183.

Richters, A. (2010). 'Community-Based Sociotherapy in Rwanda'. In Kaptegins, L. & Richters, A. (Eds.) *Mediations of Violence in Africa: Fashioning New Futures for Contested Pasts*. Leiden: Brill, pp. 74–90.

Sen, A. (1999). *Development as Freedom*. Oxford: Oxford University Press.

Saul, J. (2014). *Collective Trauma, Collective Healing: Promoting Community Resilience in the Aftermath of Disaster*. New York: Routledge.

UNHCR (2001). 'The Wall behind which Refugees can Shelter: The 1951 Geneva Convention'. *Refugees*, Vol. 2. No. 123. Retrieved on 28 May 2015 from: http://www.unhcr.org/3b5e90ea0.html.

UNHCR (2012). *The State of the World's Refugees: In Search of Solidarity*. Oxford: Oxford University Press.

UNHCR (2015). 'The 1951 Refugee Convention'. Retrieved on 28 May 2015 from: http://www.unhcr.org/pages/49da0e466.html.

Vasilevska, B. (2014). 'The Role of Settlement Agencies in Promoting Refugee Resilience'. In Simich, L. & Andermann, L. (Eds.) *Refuge and Resilience: International Perspectives on Migration*. New York: Springer, pp. 167–181.

Wanga-Odhiambo, G. (2014). *Resilience in South Sudanese Women: Hope for Daughters of the Nile*. Lanham: Lexington Books.

Zoellner, L.A. & Feeny, N.C. (2014). 'Conceptualizing Risk and Resilience Following Trauma Exposure'. In Zoellner, L.A. & Feeny, N.C. (Eds.) *Facilitating Resilience and Recovery Following Trauma*. New York: The Guilford Press, pp. 3–14.

Zolli, A. & Healy, A.M. (2012). *Resilience: Why Things Bounce Back*. New York: Free Press.

Chapter 6
Peacebuilding in South Sudan and Beyond: From Assumption to Reality

> *In the human context, peace should mean recognition of the unlimited potential buried in each and every human being, and commitment to help each other unleash the creativity in every single human being.*
> Muhammad Yunus, Sydney Peace Prize Lecture, 1998

6.1 Assuming Peace: *'You Just Assume'*

Peace is an 'assumed' state for many of the South Sudanese refugees in Kakuma. As expressed by some of the participants, this means that peace is non-existent in reality, and only seen when conjured up in one's imagination, or performed into existence. Atem used the metaphor of peace as 'an umbrella' to capture this assumption of peace:

> *Yes, I don't see there is peace there. No peace. It's a matter of an umbrella like this one* [pointing to the umbrella shade we were sitting under] *maybe if there is. Let me say for example, this umbrella, if it rains, will not protect us here, it will protect us here* [pointing above us], *and around here* [pointing to the area surrounding the umbrella], *it would still be raining on us.*[1]

Atem in effect points to the supposed appeal of peace as a concept, and its appearance of effectiveness, while in reality it seems to contain no substance. What is crucial about it is that the survivors are aware of the apparent emptiness of this assumed peace, but that does not stop them from attempting to be part of it. Juliet a 23 year old woman from the Dinka community, captures the emptiness of this peace in her expression, admitting that she had said there is peace, while in a real sense there was no peace:

> *Actually, I don't have peace. Because what I apply is in the negative, for me just to be at peace with others. But inside me, I have 'pain'. Because may be someone can mistake me. Mostly here in Sudan, like now since I don't have a husband and I'm staying with the children, someone can just come and abuse me. Someone can find me passing over there,*

[1]Interview with Atem on 2 July 2013. See Appendix 6.1.

L.W. Gitau, *Trauma-Sensitivity and Peacebuilding*, The Anthropocene: Politik—Economics—Society—Science 12, DOI 10.1007/978-3-319-49803-4_6

> *and abuse me, 'You did this to your husband that's why he left'. You see, such a thing. Now I'm not staying in peace… Now, since now there is no peace, even though I'm saying there is peace, there is no actual, there is no real peace.*[2]

This peace seems to deny the real state of things and adopt an attitude that all is well. It requires avoiding the real issue, and dwelling on the surface. It involves sacrificing one's own needs and deep-seated feelings for the sake of 'peace'. It is, as Okot, one of the participants put it, burying that 'dark stone in my stomach that somebody cannot see' and learning to 'laugh like others' and 'show my teeth' to everyone so that they believe he is happy, while he is aching inside.[3]

This peace entails going by the official construction of what needs to happen on the larger scale of things, and not concentrating on individual and community-specific needs. This kind of peace emphasizes peaceful coexistence among people from warring groups, without necessarily going deep into the issues that caused the rift between them. It is giving up one's self for the greater good. Juliet describes this peace, which first involves avoiding the conflict, and second conforming to the pre-constructed peace, which she called the 'peace that was signed':

> *What peace means to me, is that now as … we are living in this family, we try to avoid each other. When one talks badly, we have to come together and consult, and stay as brothers and sisters. Yeah, like now what happened in Sudan, there was a fight. After the fight now, they have this peace that was signed on…the peace that was signed… 2005 that was signed, yeah, that peace now, that peace is trying to bring us together and combine us together. That's what is peace according to me. Now we are staying in peace, as we are living here in the camp. We don't have conflict with some others. If someone tries to tell you something you avoid, for peace to exist.*[4]

The 'peace that was signed in 2005' refers to the Comprehensive Peace Agreement (CPA) signed on 9 January 2005 in Naivasha, Kenya, which brought to an end the Second Civil War in South Sudan (LeRiche/Arnold 2012). The CPA was supposed to usher in a period of peace in which the possibilities of either Southern Sudan uniting with, or having independence from the Sudan, would be considered. During the period following the CPA, it was assumed that there was peace in South Sudan, and UNHCR organized voluntary repatriation of South Sudanese refugees from Kakuma (UNHCR 2005).

Juliet goes on to explain this conformity to the 'official peace', the peace that is required of them as refugees in Kakuma, and how it translates to their everyday lives in the camp:

> *Like now since UNHCR and LWF insist we must have peace in the camp, now it will bring more peace if I as a person who needs peace, I help… Applying peace, may be at the water tap, when I go there and I find somebody that has taken my 'mtungi' [water container]*

[2]Interview with Juliet on 3 July 2013. See Appendix 6.1.

[3]Interview with Okot on 2 July 2013. See Appendix 6.1.

[4]Interview with Juliet on 3 July 2013. See Appendix 6.1.

> *back there, behind there and I was in position one, I will just let the person fetch water and I fetch later. That is peace.*[5]

This kind of peace that the survivors are supposed to maintain in the camp, is an example of Galtung's concept of negative peace 'where there is no [direct] violence but no other form of interaction either and where the best characterization is "peaceful coexistence"' (Galtung 1975: 29). This kind of peace, as Jeong (1999: 24) points out, emphasizes 'a stable social order', and 'does not seriously question the causes of recurring violence in existing social relations'. It is focused on the present or the near future.

The officially constructed peace that the refugees are required to keep is comparable to the official narrative of peace and reconciliation produced by truth commissions problematized by Humphrey (2002). Humphrey (2002:121) argues that truth commissions, through attempts to establish a collective memory of the atrocities experienced, in effect 'construct the sacrificial victim to expel the violence'. This way of constructing an official peace, which is supposed to act as a defense against lack of peace, and recurring violence, is in jeopardy.

If this peace simply conceals the 'nothing' void inside, if it covers the unhealed inner 'pain' described by the participants, and the invisible 'dark stone in my stomach', if it acts simply as 'an umbrella' that has the appearance of protecting everyone from the merciless rain-drops from the top, while they continue getting hopelessly wet from the sides, then it seems there is a gap that needs addressing. As seen in Chaps. 4 and 5, the survivors have gone through deep traumatic experiences, they have received various interventions to help them cope with these experiences, and some of them have portrayed notable resilience in coping with their experiences. This points to the importance of a sensitivity to the survivors' pain and trauma, an effort to fill the void with substance, a resolve to protect the survivors on all sides, in crafting a 'real' peace.

Why do the survivors continue to cling to the assumed peace? What value is there in this kind of peace? It is as though they are saying, 'Better this than nothing.' This seems to point to their desperation. Peace is so desired, that anything that seems to have the appearance of peace seems welcome.

In so far as the assumed peace translates into an imagination of peace, however, and how it can look like if it were real, the assumption of peace has great value. Peace scholars have pointed to the value of imagining peace. Philpott (2010: 9) and Lederach/Appleby (2010: 23) point to the 'utopian' idea of peace, acknowledging that peace in this mode 'may exist only in our imaginations and on paper, rather than in the real world of practice.' Lederach and Appleby see value in this kind of imagination of peace and argue that

> … an ideal-type definition offers the advantage of identifying the distance between the current scope, scale, and transformative impact of efforts to end violence and build peace, on one hand, and the fullest possible realization of peacebuilding potential, on the other (2010: 24).

[5]Interview with Juliet on 3 July 2013. See Appendix 6.1.

The argument here is that if peace can be imagined, then it can be possible, and it can eventually become real. The imagination, however, does not automatically translate to reality, but calls for certain efforts to make it concrete. Positive images of peace in the future can empower creative action that can lead to change today (Boulding 2003). With this vision, Boulding (2003: 83–93) has conducted workshops on 'Imaging a Nonviolent World' with various groups, in which she encourages participants to imagine a non-violent world in the future and describe actions they are willing to commit to doing in order to make this world a reality.

The theory and practice of Appreciative Inquiry (AI) developed by David Cooperrider and his colleagues in the mid-1980s (Liebler/Sampson 2003) speaks to the idea of imagining peace, in its emphasis on a step-by-step process of establishing a vision [of peace], and then working towards realising the vision:

> AI involves the art and practice of asking questions that strengthen a system's capacity to heighten positive potential…. In AI, intervention gives way to imagination and innovation; instead of negation, criticism and spiralling diagnosis there is discovery, dream and design. AI assumes that every living system has untapped, rich, and inspiring accounts of the positive (Cooperrider/Whitney 1999: 10, quoted in Whitney et al. 2003: 28).

The emphasis here is on the positive. In discussing the operationalization of AI, Whitney et al. (2003) point out that a focus on strengths rather than on problems, on the possibilities rather than the impracticalities, is a more effective way of realising the vision. This focus, of necessity, calls for a sensitivity to the traumatic experiences of the survivors. The vision and hope is seen to rise from an acknowledgement and appreciation of the pain and despair experienced by the survivors.

How do we go from an assumed peace to a peace in reality? Dabor, one of the participants, when asked to define peace, sadly says:

> *Yes, I understand peace, but I don't know peace. When will it be for real? ... I don't see.*[6]

What it might take to experience a 'real' peace is explored in the following sections.

6.2 Building Relationships: *'Peace Is You'*

Most participants defined peace in terms of relationships. Peace was conceived in relation to how people related with one another, in the camp and elsewhere. The concept of 'relating as brothers and sisters', which had the connotation of family, was prevalent in describing these relationships. When I asked Amuka what peace meant to her for example, she said:

> *Peace is whereby somebody or relatives, visit you, and chat together with you. And someone like a neighbour, who can show love and affection to you and that she cares. Now if something happens to you here, she can be there. That's when I can realise that there is*

[6]Interview with Dabor on 16 July 2013. See Appendix 6.1.

peace. But if there is nothing like that, I don't know where peace goes, or where peace comes from... the peace that I can see is you. Like now you've come to visit me and interview me and before you came here, no one has ever visited me. I just stay here lonely. I stay here with the children, and even no one can realise that this woman is suffering from this and that.[7]

Amuka connected the subject of loneliness to peace. For her, there can be no peace if one is lonely. Connection with others, friends, family and neighbours, is what creates peace. She saw value in the interview for this reason.

The idea of a shared community life, with give and take undertones, seemed to prevail in the participants' description of peace. Peace is something shared. Fazila called it 'a two way traffic' whereby 'I have to give you peace, and you also have to give me peace'.[8] Riek said:

Peace, I have to begin by myself... I myself I must have the confidence to have peace. I have to respect myself, before I give respect to anyone... Second, I have to show peace, by the way I interact with people, the way I talk to them, the way I help the community, it means peace. I must show by example first... After that, I will be in position to bring peace to the community.[9]

Peace as described by these participants entails self-reflection, but even then, the self-reflection is in relation to how they examine themselves in order to relate with others in more constructive ways. Samir described this self-reflection, leading to constructive relationships, hence peace, this way:

Personally I'll start peace within myself by recognising myself first. I should recognize the person I am, and be contented...That I am that person. Weak or strong, rich or poor, I should be contented that I am that person. So, after having recognized myself, then surely I'm also going to recognize the person next to me. I'll value his dignity, or her dignity, and I have already valued mine. So when I valued mine and I value hers or his. Then there I'm sure there is no conflict between me and that person.[10]

Peace as a quiet, private, tranquil undisturbed state is a foreign concept for the survivors. Interdependence rather than independence marks a peaceful society. No one wanted to be left alone to muse over his or her misfortunes in solitude. When they suffered, they gathered.

'Bringing peace to the community', as Riek[11] called it, entails reaching out to those in need, giving a helping hand. Pubudu put it this way:

Peace is a... is like you now. When you see those with problems and can go to help them... you can help them to become good. Or if there is somebody looking... or in the community ... you can go and ask them what is the problem, and you can help them.[12]

[7]Interview with Amuka on 3 July 2013. See Appendix 6.1.

[8]Interview with Fazila on 5 July 2013. See Appendix 6.1.

[9]Interview with Riek on 11 July 2013. See Appendix 6.1.

[10]Interview with Samir on 8 July 2013. See Appendix 6.1.

[11]Interview with Riek on 11 July 2013. See Appendix 6.1.

[12]Interview with Pubudu on 5 July 2013. See Appendix 6.1.

With these words and throughout the interview, Pubudu implied that I, as the interviewer, should help him and others 'acquire peace' by helping them out with their material needs. This means that those who are financially able are seen to have the responsibility of meeting the needs of those who are not.

Even in terms of education, which the participants cited as a most important intervention, the idea of other-centredness and a community orientation recurs. In describing his attempts to solicit for the building of a library for the young people of his church community, Jerem for example, saw no value in anything that would benefit him alone, as an individual, and said, 'My heart is for everyone and I think everyone could be assisted, not me alone …'[13]

Atem's story illustrates the value of relationships, in envisioning a future of peace. Atem assists others by being involved in leadership opportunities in his community, and sees peace as comprising of living in harmony with both his fellow refugees and the host community, the Turkana people who neighbour the camp. He says:

> *Here in Kakuma, we live together in peace, even with the host community, the Turkana. We live as good neighbours, brothers and sisters, and share water and food. I try to maintain peace with them, and with their leader, the DO (District Officer).*[14]

Fazila[15] considers the opportunities she has received to further her education, including going for university studies in Canada, as an opportunity to reach out to others in her community and to facilitate peace. She hopes to go back to her country after her studies and contribute to the peacebuilding process.

Riek[16] depends on the elders in his community for counsel and support in his role as the tribal leader of his community. He also seeks support from his friends and neighbours who are married, to help him fulfill his responsibilities as a leader. At the time of the interview, Riek was involved in reconciliation efforts between his tribe, the Nuer, and the Murle tribe who had clashed in the camp. He also hopes to be involved in peacebuilding processes back in South Sudan in the future.

Patrick[17] is similarly involved in the reconciliation efforts between his tribe the Murle, and the Nuer in the camp. He also sees his work as a livestock officer, in which he encourages the community to desist from cattle-raiding, a major source of conflict and violence between tribes in South Sudan. He depends on other members of the community for support in his roles. Similarly, Grace[18] depends on her support group of fellow HIV positive colleagues and the counsellor for support, and seeks and values the company of her friends and neighbours who occasionally

---

[13]Interview with Jerem on 13 July 2013. See Appendix 6.1.

[14]Interview with Atem on 2nd July 2013. See Appendix 6.1.

[15]Interview with Fazilla, 5th July 2013. See Appendix 6.1.

[16]Interview with Riek on 11th July 2013. See Appendix 6.1.

[17]Interview with Patrick on 15th and 16th July 2013. See Appendix 6.1.

[18]Interview with Grace on 17th July 2013. See Appendix 6.1.

come to visit. She is also seen to reach out to others through her support of her deceased brother's family.

Peace as relationship also involves diversity. There are people from different nationalities in Kakuma, and as such, they have to interact with each other and learn to live with one another, as Samir explained in defining peace:

> *...now this camp is full of diversity... And wherever you move, apart from your home, once you get out of this gate, of this compound, I have to meet people from different points of the world. So there, when I meet a person of such kind, I have to abandon my own, or hide my own personality first and try to study his personality. After studying his personality, I'll now put my shoe or admit myself into his or hers. So he will surely find that I am concerned with his or her affairs... And he will also develop some liking for me. So we'll come to be together and have no grudges against each other. Which is already peace.*[19]

This interconnectedness that the participants described in their definitions of peace is indicative of Martin Buber's 'I-Thou' approach (Buber 1922) discussed in Chap. 3 as the underlying philosophy of the discussion of the concept of peace in this study. Buber envisioned a community in which individuals have essentially to do with one another, but at the same time the personal life of all is enriched and not diminished. The individual is not subsumed in the community, but rather, recognizes his or her personhood by recognising the uniqueness and otherness of the other person—realising that one would never be able to use the terminology 'I' if there did not exist a 'You' to contrast it with. A person's very nature, his or her personhood, is embedded in the other person, which has transforming power. This transforming encounter is what we find in the composite character Talia, in Chap. 1, when she realizes the fusion between herself and her supposed enemy and hands her shoes over to him.

This concept of interconnectedness resonates with the African philosophy of Ubuntu, which similarly conceives personhood in relation to others (Gade 2013). Ubuntu is the essence of being human. The spirit of Ubuntu is captured for instance in Xhosa, one of South African's official languages, as *Umntu ngumntu ngabanye abantu* which translated into English is 'People are people through other people' (Chaplin n.d). In tracing the West African concept of peace for example, Opoku (2014: 418) points to the emphasis on community which is born of an awareness of the interdependence of people. With this regard, the West African proverb: 'The left hand washes the right and the right hand washes the left' (Opoku 2014: 418) aptly captures this interconnectedness of people. Gebrewold (2014: 428) similarly discusses the Eastern African perspective of peace from the vantage point of the Kambaata people of Ethiopia, who have a similar saying as the South African people: *Mannu manna ihanohu manninet*, which when translated into English means, 'A person becomes a person through fellow persons.' The word for peace in Kambaata language is *t'úmmu,* which is an all-encompassing word denoting goodness, wellness, kindness, generosity, and justice. Gebrewold (2014: 430–431) discusses the major ways of maintaining or creating peace which include greetings

---

[19]Interview with Samir on 8 July 2013. See Appendix 6.1.

and feasts, which entail sharing in each other's joys and sorrows. 'To be means to be in the community and to be in the community to be in peace', Gebrewold (2014: 431) concludes. Similarly, in the Kiswahili language which is spoken in most parts of East and Central Africa, the word for greetings is *salamu,* derived from the Arabic word *salaam* meaning peace. The word is rich in implication of the importance of the welfare of the other person. Peace, thus, is seen as relationship.

Lederach conceptualized the essence of peacebuilding as lying in this interconnectedness of people, or what he calls a 'web of relationship' (Lederach 2005: 34–35). Understanding the dynamics and potentials of this web, and tapping into them, is seen as crucial to peacebuilding. Schirch (2004) and Jeong (2005), similarly identify the transformation of relationships as the core of peacebuilding.

The participants' identification of peace as chiefly comprised in relationships, and the main effect of their trauma as the damage to relationships, points to the symbiotic relationship that links the building of relationships with the healing of trauma. As Schirch (2004: 46–47) points out, trauma healing is one of the key interrelated processes necessary for the building of relationships, along with transforming conflict and doing justice. Similarly, trauma healing depends on building relationships and reconnecting people (Herman 1997; Schirch 2004). Gobodo-Madikizela (2008: 173) emphasizes the value of forgiveness which she argues serves 'to re-animate the empathic sensibilities damaged by violence both between individuals and within communities.' In discussing the importance of relationships in recovery from trauma, Herman (1997: 133) argues:

> Recovery can take place only within the context of relationships; it cannot occur in isolation. In her renewed connections with other people, the survivor re-creates the psychological faculties that were damaged or deformed by the traumatic experience. The faculties include the basic capacities for trust, autonomy, initiative, competence, identity, and intimacy. Just as these capabilities are originally formed in relationships with other people, they must be reformed in such relationships.

A focus on relationships leads to the idea of a community orientation in relation to envisioning and working towards peace. Peacebuilding scholars point to the opportunities that exist in relationships, especially in terms of participatory approaches and community mobilization, allowing for the tapping into the knowledge and resources of the community, and enhancing local ownership of the peacebuilding process. Kantowitz/Riak (2008: 9–10) further note:

> Participatory approaches empower communities with decision-making capacity regarding their future, in this way giving individuals and communities agency and changing the dynamic of powerlessness and an orientation towards survival that may characterize traumatized communities.

Jeong (2005: 34) similarly agues for these participatory approaches, which he refers to as 'endogenous measures', locally owned approaches that originate from the people directly affected by the conflict. Jeong contrasts these measures with 'exogenous measures, which depend on initiatives prescribed, induced, or imposed externally or from the top' (Jeong 2005: 34).

Chupp (2003) emphasizes the power of local ownership of peacebuilding projects, nested in community mobilization. He gives a case example of a group of villagers in the Usulutan province of El Salvador who came together and formed a grassroots organization to overcome violence and teach peace. They initiated their own home-grown Culture of Peace Program, developing community circles for rediscovering nonviolent problem-solving methods in their culture, and eventually declared themselves a 'Local Zone of Peace' (Chupp 2003: 96).

It appears that for the survivors, the connections with people, in the aftermath of conflict and violence, restores faith in humanity that may have been destroyed. If they can connect again to others, and work together, then there is hope for the future. The significance of the connections is made all the more poignant by the state of separation, disappearance and death of loved ones that the survivors are still working to live with. According to the participants, relationships, built on the foundation of inner self-reflection, form the core of peace.

6.3 An Inclusive Peace: *'Peace Is Everything'*

Some of the participants had a wider perception of peace and understood it to entail broader issues that impacted on their lives. This wider perception included considering and addressing the issues that had led to the destruction of peace in the first place, including political issues, structural inequalities, land and cattle disputes, and tribal enmities. Chriz articulated some of these issues in his definition of peace:

> *Peace is the absence of war and other conflicts. If there's no war and the other conflicts, it's like war may stop but other conflicts may continue, like leadership wrangles in the government and the other conflicts like cattle rustling in the country, and other conflicts.*[20]

Peace is seen to involve more than the absence of war, though the absence of war and armed conflict are its lowest common denominator (Akerlund 2005). Absence of war in this case means not only the absence of physical violence, but psychological violence as well, including what Patrick called 'psychological conflict',[21] or war directed towards the other person's psyche, with the aim of demoralising them. In defining peace, Patrick explained it means:

> *... when people live a whole life, complete life, where there is no fighting, or hatred that we are talking about, or conflict physical or psychological conflict.*[22]

[20]Interview with Chriz on 10 July 2013. See Appendix 6.1.

[21]It is important here to note that in many African languages, including the *Murle* dialect that Patrick speaks, the same word is used for both 'conflict' and 'war', hence Patrick, though he spoke in English in the interview, directly translated the word as conflict. In another instance, he referred to the same issue as 'psychological war, to injure you', as quoted in Chap. 4.

[22]Interview with Patrick on 15 and 16 July 2013. See Appendix 6.1.

Patrick described the ways in which psychological war had been waged against his community by other tribes, who referred to his tribe as 'rebels' and 'worthless'.[23]

In her definition of peace, Fazila referred to the all-inclusiveness of peace in these words:

> *Peace means a lot. Peace is everything. Peace, I know in simpler terms it's the absence of war. So when there is peace, you know there is a lot of development. Development in terms of economy, you know, people living together, loving one another, so peace is actually very important. Because there will be no death, there will be education, you know people will be able to establish may be schools to study, and there will be a lot of development. So peace is actually good.*[24]

These all-inclusive aspects of peace are incorporated in the concept of positive peace, as defined by Galtung (1976) and Jeong (1999), involving the structural, cultural and political attributes. Galtung sees peace as very directly related to the fulfilment of the four classes of basic needs, namely survival needs, well-being needs, identity needs and freedom needs. He argues that the negation of survival needs would mean 'death and mortality', the absence of well-being needs would lead to 'misery and morbidity', the negation of identity needs leads to alienation, and the absence of freedom to repression (Galtung 1996: 197). Jeong (1999: 25) similarly embraces this broad understanding of peace and sees the goals of positive peace as touching upon issues that influence the quality of life, including 'personal growth, freedom, social equality, economic equity, solidarity, autonomy and participation.' This understanding is in line with Patrick's definition of peace as living 'a whole life, complete life', and Fazila's description of peace as 'everything'.

Peace involves security. As Rita pointed out in her definition, peace meant she could feel safe, and not in danger of sudden violent attack, as she had experienced in South Kordofan before fleeing for safety in the camp:

> *Peace means to stay free in your home, without any fear, and without any attack... day or night, and without any bombing of antonovs and bombing of helicopters. That's what peace means.*[25]

Security as it pertains to peace entails human security, comprising of 'freedom from fear' and 'freedom from want' (Hayes/Mason 2013: 4–5). This second aspect of peace comprises the basic necessities of food, shelter, and health facilities. Provision of basic necessities comprised the main intervention the refugees said they received in the camp.

Related to security is the concept of freedom. In addition to freedom from want in terms of the basic necessities, this concept entails freedom from threat and any form of harassment. This is especially in relation to women who felt threatened and

[23]See a discussion of 'psychological war' in relation to dehumanization and its effect in Chap. 4.

[24]Interview with Fazila on 5 July 2013. See Appendix 6.1.

[25]Interview with Rita on 4 July 2013. See Appendix 6.1.

had faced sexual and domestic violence as a consequence of the conflict, as expressed by Joy:

> *Peace is the state of being secure. It's a process of being safe and secure from any kind of violence. Yeah. Any kind of violence. That includes... Like harassment, assault, threat.*[26]

The breakdown of culture and the resultant erosion of cultural values and social cohesion had left many survivors vulnerable and insecure. They lacked the family and community support that had characterized their lives before displacement in the camp. Further, freedom entails being able to make choices and have control of one's own life, an aspect that is lacking in the refugee camp. As discussed in Chap. 4, the refugees' dependence on UNHCR disrupted the crucial dynamic of a sense of control over their lives. In defining peace therefore, Matida described it as a state of freedom, being able to 'do what you know'.[27]

Another crucial aspect of positive peace is citizenship. The sense of lack of belonging is one of the major marks of the refugee experience. Many participants talked longingly about belonging to a country, and some talked nostalgically about their 'motherland', hoping to go back there some day. In defining peace, Zeneb contrasted the state of fear and uncertainty the South Sudanese refugees were in, with the citizenship Kenyans were enjoying:

> *Like now in Kenya, there is a positive peace, 'cause they are now well settled, and each and every one, each and every citizen believes they are in their country. But in Southern Sudan, I've seen we still fear.*[28]

Peace then is the sense of a home, a place, where the refugees can stay, without being sent away, where the law protects them and gives them some form of stability, as Paulo put it:

> *Peace is whereby people stay together. People like now in the camp, we can say that they have peace why, because they are there in their houses, and nothing can chase them away from there... no one can tell us, 'Now you move from this place, go!' There is peace. We can stay. That's what I understand.*[29]

In *The Origins of Totalitarianism*, Arendt (1994) talks about political citizenship as a major requirement of one's sense of humanness. If one does not belong to a political entity, he or she is lost as a human being. If there is no one to claim the person politically, then it is as though he or she does not exist. Without citizenship, the other aspects such as security, freedom and development do not hold. Arendt (1994: 299–300) says of a person stripped of his or her citizenship:

> … it seems that a man who is nothing but a man has lost the very qualities which make it possible for other people to treat him as a fellow-man… the world found nothing sacred in the abstract nakedness of being human.

---

[26]Interview with Joy on 16 July 2013. See Appendix 6.1.

[27]Interview with Matida on 4 July 2013. See Appendix 6.1.

[28]Interview with Zeneb on 3 July 2013. See Appendix 6.1.

[29]Interview with Paulo on 3 July 2013. See Appendix 6.1.

Here, Arendt is pointing to the stark reality of things. Though we know a human being is of value in and of himself or herself, and we have seen how this value extends in relation to others, the reality of things is that politically, one still needs to belong somewhere, duly registered and officially recognized, in order to enjoy certain rights.

Reychler (2001: 12) refers to the all-encompassing concept of peace discussed in this section as 'sustainable peace', which he defines as:

> …a situation characterized by the absence of physical violence, the elimination of unacceptable political, economic, and cultural forms of discrimination; a high level of internal and external legitimacy or support; self-sustainability, and propensity to enhance the constructive transformation of conflicts.

Omeje (2013) points to this all-inclusiveness of peace in discussing the diversity and complexity of conflict in the African Great Lakes region. Human security, safety from direct, structural and cultural violence, and justice, are all key to peacebuilding after mass violence.

This kind of peace requires a wide array of actors, working synergetically to ensure a holistic approach to peacebuilding that will comprehensively tackle the various aspects, entailing what Lederach (1997: 20) refers to as 'the full array of processes, approaches, and stages needed to transform conflict toward more sustainable, peaceful relationships.'

While the factors described in this section may be considered the outer characteristics of peace, their presence or lack thereof is experienced and expressed in terms of the survivors' inner perceptions and relationships, as seen in the participants' descriptions, and discussed in the previous section on 'Building Relationships'. This points to the interconnectedness of inner and outer peace. In the next section we will explore how this inner and outer peace can be developed together as a 'real' peace that goes beyond the assumed or imagined peace discussed at the beginning of this chapter.

6.4 Creating Possibilities: *'I Developed Courage'*

This section discusses the possibilities of creating a real peace, that exists in the participants' perceptions of peace and their experiences. These possibilities are seen in the participants' expressions of hope and courage, an integrated approach of interventions, and a creative approach to their experiences.

6.4.1 Hope and Courage

Some participants expressed hope despite what they had suffered back in South Sudan, on the journey to the camp, and in the camp. Atem for instance described how he was hopeful for a better life, despite his past experiences and present circumstances:

> *Yes I'm hopeful. On my side I'm hopeful because I tried. I lost all the parents, even my brothers and sisters... I forget the past. And now I'm starting the new life. Yes.*[30]

Joy explained that she had developed 'the courage that I can do like any other person', and acted on this courage with the attitude that despite the circumstances surrounding her, a better life was possible. She said:

> *OK. Me I think life is not that very bad in the camp. 'Cause there is no way that you can be totally in a very bad situation without any help. We have a lot of services and structures that can help.*[31]

Other participants expressed faith and hope in God. They believe it is possible to make it in life, and that it is possible to find peace. Jean Paul expressed this faith by saying:

> *My hope here in the camp is, you know, everything is God, You don't know what God will make you to be. Because God knows what to do...*[32]

This expression of hope by the participants resonates with the discipline of paradoxical curiosity in Lederach's (2005) concept of the moral imagination discussed in Chap. 3. Paradoxical curiosity is the ability to 'rise above dualistic polarities' (Lederach 2005: 36). It involves an appreciation and respect for the complexity of issues in the conflict context, and allowing for multiple and even contradictory social realities. The most common picture of the refugee, which exists as a result of the image constructed by the humanitarian industry (Butt 2002; Humphrey 2002) is one of a helpless, dependent individual in need of rescue. As seen in this hope and courage expressed by the survivors, and in the discussion on resilience however, a number of participants showed that they do not fit into the category of the helpless, dependent, suffering refugee who must be rescued. There is potential in these participants to rise above the conventional image of the suffering, helpless refugee as it were, and be productive.

The hope and courage can further be seen as what Lederach (2005) describes as the willingness to take a risk, in his theory of the moral imagination. This involves stepping with courage into the unknown without having an assurance that things will turn out well. The faith in God and hope expressed by the participants is a risk in itself. 'Faith is the assurance of things hoped for; the certainty of things not seen', as the Bible says in Hebrews 11:1. The survivors, in their faith, take a risk by hoping for and believing in what they have not seen.

Despite what has happened, the losses experienced and destruction witnessed, one can still move on with life and hope for peace. In his book *Passion for Peace*, Rees (2003: 39–41) underscores the importance of 'overcoming fatalism' and the

---

[30]Interview with Atem on 2 July 2013. See Appendix 6.1.

[31]Interview with Joy on 16 July 2013. See Appendix 6.1.

[32]Interview with Jean Paul on 15 July 2013. See Appendix 6.1.

possibility of rediscovering optimism even in the grimmest of situations. In discussing the risk that may be called for in imagining and acting towards the reality of peace, Audergon says:

> Considering all the violence in our world, it is natural to feel a sense of despair or hopelessness. But, can we dare to imagine taking responsibility for our history and future? … Can we find ways to include the tragedy and traumas of our personal and collective history into our hearts without repeating them? Can we imagine a world where we actively work with the history and conflicts from which we suffer, rather than fall into repeating them? (2008: 261–262).

Audergon (2008) gives an example of a project in which she and her colleagues 'dared to dream' about transforming a most difficult situation, by bringing together Croats, Serbs and Muslims for the first time in Osijek, Croatia, to discuss ways of building a sustainable community in the aftermath of the war.

Again here, the theory of Appreciative Inquiry resonates with the idea of hope and courage expressed by the participants, and the risk involved. Liebler/Sampson (2003) view the inquiry as a journey into the unknown, and an imagining of the possible. They argue:

> This journey involves improvization and a certain amount of risk. It begins with a general vision of the direction and an idea of the type of trip you're embarking on, but leaves a lot of room for the unexpected to happen along the way (Liebler/Sampson 2003: 56).

The 'general vision' is the assumed peace described in the first section, and the 'unexpected' are the possibilities presented in this section in relation to hope, courage and creativity.

Whitney et al. (2003) embrace the idea of moving forward in courage and taking a risk in envisioning trauma healing for trauma survivors using the concept of Appreciative Inquiry. The risk entails 'remembering of strengths and capacities, a recollection or re-creation of dreams, and a reclaiming of identity in community'(Whitney et al. 2003: 49–50).

Sider (2003: 287) takes this further, proposing the use of 'appreciative interviewing' as a specific tool for discovering and retrieving stories that expand the language of hope and enhance the pursuit of healing and growth for the survivors. This tool helps in identifying resources to transcend trauma. Sider argues:

> In the field of trauma healing and recovery, the appreciative interview – the Discovery Phase of Appreciative Inquiry (AI) – can awaken and uncover positive healing forces. Appreciative interviewing involves the art and science of asking questions that strengthen people's capacities to tap into and heighten their positive potential (Cooperrider et al. 2000). If people move in the direction of the questions they ask and where they consistently focus attention, then … Questions employing a vocabulary of hope, on the other hand, can direct attention to the possibilities for healing and growth that exist in the midst of loss. This type of questioning begins to shine light on – to uncover or reveal – positive and restorative processes that exist but might not otherwise be seen (Sider 2003: 293).

The participants' stories attest to the potential that exists in asking questions that direct attention to the possibilities for recovery from trauma and restoration of capacities for engagement in productive activities, while acknowledging and appreciating the pain and desperation experienced by the survivors.

6.4.2 Education and Integration

Education was one of the most quoted intervention by the refugees, alongside the basic services of food, shelter, medication and security. In describing the power that education has to transform, Fazila, said:

> *... education has actually changed me personally. And so, you know, education is important because it will actually help you one day may be to be able to you know, be of some help to the problem, or try to solve the problem that people are experiencing,... may be try to stop the war, you know. Education is power. I think these people, most people are not educated, that's why they are just fighting.*[33]

Fazila thus connects the conflict and mass violence that has resulted in the survivors' displacement with lack of education. Patrick similarly makes this connection when he says:

> *I think one of the problems causing conflict is lack of education. So we want people who have already come here to get educated, so that when, maybe in future they go back, they will be able to solve their problems in a good way.*[34]

Education is thus seen by the participants as a gateway to peace. As such, it can be integrated with other interventions to help the survivors work through their traumatic experiences and be involved in building peace. Education for instance may be co-opted to help deal with the psychological aftermath of traumatic experiences (Staub et al. 2008). Staub and colleagues developed an educational approach to promote healing and reconciliation in Rwanda in the aftermath of the genocide. The approach aimed to educate participants in understanding the effects of trauma and victimization and avenues of healing, discuss the roots of genocide, understand basic psychological needs, and engage with the experience of the genocide and share stories with each other (Staub et al. 2008: 135–137).

This kind of integration can also be adapted to other interventions alongside education. The integration demonstrates a sensitivity to the survivors' differing realities. Vasilevska's (2014) four principles, which she derived from her study examining the role of agencies in supporting the settlement and resilience of refugees can be used to inform this integration. These include *complexity, decentrality, atypicality* and cultural *relativity*. *Complexity* entails adapting a holistic

---

[33]Interview with Fazila on 5 July 2013. See Appendix 6.1.

[34]Interview with Patrick on 15 and 16 July 2013. See Appendix 6.1.

integrated approach and not a narrowly defined one in the interventions (Vasilevska 2014: 169), as discussed above with regard to education integrating a focus on trauma healing.

Decentrality refers to aligning different services so that the various needs of the survivors are not met in isolation from each other, but rather together. A problem with shelter, for instance, may be interconnected with domestic violence and issues of health, as happened to be the case with Sara.[35] Sara had run to the camp reception centre seeking shelter, but it emerged that she was escaping domestic violence from her 'co-wife', had a dysfunctional relationship with her husband, and suffered mental health issues. Attention to her problem with shelter would entail sensitivity to her family situation and her mental health, including the progression and presentation of her symptoms which, as discussed in Chap. 5, appear to be a way of re-legitimizing herself as a person of worth.

Atypicality involves going outside the box and taking a radical perspective which is oriented towards the survivor, not on the way something would be typically done (Vasilevska 2014). This for instance may involve challenging the image of the refugee as a helpless person, incapable of offering support. For instance, asking the refugees to contribute towards helping someone else who needs support, or to support the person offering the intervention in some way, goes against the typical way refugees are viewed and may challenge their own outlook of themselves as helpless. Zeneb, one of the participants of this research who was born and orphaned in the camp, became my self-appointed research assistant during my fieldwork in Kakuma, and in this role portrayed initiative and competence.

Cultural relativity entails acknowledging and being sensitive to different cultural values in the interventions (Vasilevska 2014: 178). This may involve a sensitivity to the ways in which the refugees' cultural values have been eroded as a consequence of the displacement to the camp. Joy for instance related how the women in her community had turned to brewing illicit beer as a result of the 'men's irresponsibility'. Traditionally in South Sudan, men are supposed to provide for their families, but in the camp, the UNHCR and its partnering agencies provide for all the refugees, rendering men's role impotent hence their supposed 'irresponsibility'. This sensitivity may lead to withholding judgement in response to the situation, as well as carefully considering the appropriateness of an intervention in this case, and thinking of alternative ways for men to express their 'responsibility'.

In its appreciation of the complexity of the survivors' experiences, this integration of services seeks to uphold the respect for all people as individuals, and protect human dignity. It entails what the psychologist Carl Rogers referred to as 'Unconditional Positive Regard' (UPR) (Rogers 1961: 283), which means accepting and respecting others as they are without judgement or evaluation.

---

[35]Interview with Sara on 4 July 2013. See Appendix 6.1.

6.4.3 Creativity

The creative approach to the participants' experience involves going beyond what is experienced or expressed, while speaking to it at the same time, as is the nature of poetry, fine art, music and creative writing (Lederach 2005: 38). For this reason, here I do not present what the participants said with regard to creativity, but rather draw inferences about how what they said suggests the need for such creativity, building on the insights of peace scholars. One of the most poignant expressions that shows the need for this creativity is Okot's expression in describing his experience in the camp:

> *When there is no way, you just keep quiet.*[36]

The 'nothing' and 'just staying' themes discussed in Chap. 4, whereby we see the participants resigned to whatever may happen to them, also show the need for this approach, as does the empty distant look that many of the participants I interviewed wore.

The phrase 'going beyond what is experienced' is apt here because the experiences of some of the survivors in this study seem inconceivable and may not be readily and literally expressible. In her book *Ritual and Symbol in Peacebuilding*, Schirch (2005) discusses the power of ritual and symbolic acts in transforming relationships in situations of conflict and violence. She points out that since symbols communicate indirectly, they are able to communicate a message with more than one interpretation. Rituals and symbols are part of life, and as such, can naturally be harnessed to speak to the crucial process of peacebuilding. Van der Merwe/Vienings (2001: 344) also point to the value of rituals in dealing with collective traumas, for example rituals helping communities to deal with the past through remembering people who have died and the loss the community has suffered.

The use of humour is one creative means of dealing with extreme situations such as war and conflict as 'it reveals the twistedness of the situation, and in so doing upholds the human capacity to understand and survive even the incomprehensible' (Williams 2001: 492). Humour helps to facilitate the adaptation to a difficult situation, helps to displace and channel other emotions such as anger and despair which if allowed would enhance the survivor's vulnerability, helps to socialize and reassert one's humanity in the face of the inhuman, and helps to convey the truth safely (Williams 2001: 492–494).

In discussing the use of the arts in peacebuilding, Lederach (2003: 122) points out:

> The single greatest challenge facing positive approaches to peacebuilding is found in the paradox of how people in an ongoing violent conflict can develop unexpected creative action, while living in the grips of genuine tragedy, deep injustice, oppression, and trauma.

---

[36]Interview with Okot on 2 July 2013. See Appendix 6.1.

Ayindo (2008: 185) similarly argues that the 'arts approaches to peace' have contributed to the depth of learning that is essential in response to the deep pain and trauma experienced in situations of conflict and mass violence where intervention requires more holistic approaches. Arts are part of everyday life and 'bear potential to fully challenge our imagination in search for creative, viable and sustainable alternatives' (Ayindo 2008: 186). They are of particularly crucial importance in times of pain when approaches that go beyond conventional language may be called for, because pain tends to destroy language (Scarry 1985: 232). As Hastrup (2003: 312) argues, destruction of language easily leads to destruction of the subject which language is attempting to capture, and hence the need to employ the arts to reinstate meaning into the experiences of the survivors. This reinstating of meaning leads to a sense of purpose and forms part of recovery from trauma.

Not only are some of the experiences inexpressible, they also render work and other activities difficult, if not impossible. As earlier discussed, the traumatic experiences tend to sap the energies of the survivors and leave them in no state to engage in work-related experience. The creative act could help restore the vital energies to enable the survivors to engage in meaningful activities.

The culture of the South Sudanese people that is rich in dance, music, poetry and drama has been co-opted in some instances to help develop ways that can be used to express the experiences of the survivors. Amollo (2008) discusses the transformative potential of stage drama and artistic dance, as exemplified by a project organized by the Amani Peoples Theatre (APT) in Kakuma. Regarding the power of theatre, Amollo (2008: 11) argues:

> Theatre offers the opportunity to dramatize possibilities where none existed before. It offers a space in which to try alternative ideas for resolving conflict and to jar ourselves and others loose from the spell of structural imbalances, breaking the action/reaction cycle so typical of protracted conflicts. It offers a space for exposing the offending scripts of violence and structural domination and then the ability to rewrite those scripts, enacting a drama that replaces the existing conflicts with a formula that is more human and just. In this sense, theatre becomes an active process of revision and re-enactment of the systemic structure of life.

In 'exposing the offending scripts' and the rewriting of desired scripts lies the power of transformation and the possibility of moving from an assumption of peace to a real peace.

If a community already has ritual resources for peace within its traditions, then it makes sense for peacebuilders to help the community to further develop these resources for itself (Schirch 2005: 52). The option to co-opt culture in the creativity discipline creates many opportunities to remould relationships and create community consensus (Senehi/Byrne 2011: 399). The Transcultural Psychosocial Organization (TPO), an international organization working with South Sudanese refugees in Northern Uganda since 1994 (Baron 2002), is an example of co-option of culture in peacebuilding. The TPO seeks to offer culturally sensitive psychosocial and mental health services to the refugees. It aims to not only assist individuals, families and groups cope with crisis situations, but develop long-term, self-sustainable, community-based ways of coping. It draws from the South

Sudanese culture through understanding and contextualising traditional practices related to mental health issues, training and utilising South Sudanese psychosocial counsellors, and working with traditional South Sudanese healers.

The creative approach rests on one of the key assumptions of peacebuilding, that conflict is not necessarily negative, but possesses a creative force that can be tapped for positive outcomes through the exploration of new options (Abu-Nimer 2003). As with imagining peace, the theory and practice of Appreciative Inquiry also speaks to the notion of creativity, especially in regard to the constructionist and poetic principles (Liebler/Sampson 2003). The constructionist principle of AI holds that 'we create what we can imagine', and 'we collectively make meaning of our world based on our habits, traditions, teachings, and how we view our very identity' (Liebler/Sampson 2003: 58). The poetic principle holds that 'a people's past, present, and future are endless sources of learning, inspiration, interpretation, and possibility' (Liebler/Sampson 2003: 59). The creative discipline thus takes us beyond the impossible, the imagined, to the possible.

In strengthening their hope and courage, respecting the complexity of their experiences, reconstructing their visions and dreams, and in envisioning and dreaming a peaceful future, the survivors might be helped to fill the 'nothing' void, remove the 'dark stone in the stomach', and address the deep 'pain' inside, enhancing the possibility of a 'real' peace.

6.5 Conclusion

Considering the perception of peace as an assumed state for many of the South Sudanese refugees in Kakuma, and the various ways this 'assumed peace' is experienced by different participants, there appears to be potential value that exists in this assumed state of peace, insofar as it translates into an imagination of peace as the participants would desire it.

Relationships emerge as the core of peacebuilding, as defined and discussed by the participants, in the second section. The participants' interview responses, show the value of relationships with regard to peace. Martin Buber's 'I-Thou' concept as well as the concept of Ubuntu, and other perspectives of peace in Africa, underscore the centrality of relationships in conceptualising peace. Further, a connection between relationships and the recovery from trauma, as well as the potential of peacebuilding that exists in the interconnectedness of people, emerges.

Thirdly, the all-inclusive nature of peace as presented by some participants, which entails safety from direct, structural and cultural violence, human security, and freedom is revealed. These aspects resonate with Galtung's (1975) concept of positive peace. This all-inclusiveness of peace highlights the need for an application of a holistic approach to peacebuilding that can comprehensively tackle the different aspects of both inner and outer peace.

Finally, in considering the possibilities of building a real peace that may exist in the participants' experiences, perceptions and interventions, we find opportunities to go beyond the expected, the impossible, and the unknown, that lie in the hope and courage expressed, an appreciation of the complexity of their experiences, an integration of the interventions they receive, and a creative approach in responding to their experiences. Lederach's (2005) theory of the moral imagination, as well as the theory of Appreciative Inquiry and discussions by other peace scholars shed light on these possibilities.

Appendix 6.1

Pseudonym	M/F	Ethnic group	Age	Duration of stay in the camp	Brief details	Date of interview
Grace	F	Acholi	40	14 years	Father and brother tortured and killed on being suspected to be traitors. Raped and forced into marriage by a soldier. Has given birth 14 times and only one child has survived. Also taking care of 10 of her deceased brothers' children. Was diagnosed HIV positive in the camp and resettlement process stalled. Cooks food for sale to supplement the ration in the camp	17th July 2013
Patrick	M	Murle	40	5 months	People from the Nuer Community attacked his village and killed many people, his wife and children ran to the bush where his wife delivered their last child. SPLA soldiers attacked his village, many people were killed and he sustained injuries. Worked as a Livestock officer. In the Reconciliation committee between the Murle and the Nuer in the camp	15th and 16th July 2013
Joy	F	Acholi	32	12 years	Fled civil war in South Sudan and came to camp with cousin. Mother joined her in 2003. Was unable to complete secondary education in the camp. Case worker with LWF Peacebuilding unit. Has two children and is expecting a third in a month's time. Separated from her husband	16th July 2013

(continued)

(continued)

Pseudonym	M/F	Ethnic group	Age	Duration of stay in the camp	Brief details	Date of interview
Dabor	F	Didinga	46	20 years	Escaped war between the North and the South. Parents and husband died in the war. Feared her children would be recruited as child soldiers and fled. Remarried in Kakuma, got two other children and second husband also died in the war when he went back to fight. Was working as a midwife in Kakuma hospital but lost her job in 1999. Cooks doughnuts to sell in the camp	16th July 2013
Fazila	F	Nuba	21	14 years	Family escaped due to the war between South Sudan and Arabs in 1999. Came to the camp with step-mother and two siblings. Father an SPLA. Mother joined them in the camp in 2012. Has won scholarship and is preparing to go to University in Canada in August	5th July 2013
Zeneb	F	Dinka	20	20 years	Born in the camp. Father went back to South Sudan in 1996 and was short dead. Moved to Nairobi with mother in 2003 to attend school. Mother died in 2010 as a result of wounds sustained in the post-election violence in Kenya in 2008. Working as an incentive case worker with Peacebuilding unit of LWF	3rd July 2013
Riek	M	Nuer	27	8 years	Escaped due to insecurity after his parents, fiancée and unborn child died. Has taken advantage of different education opportunities in the camp. Works as a community leader. Involved in reconciliation efforts between the Nuer and the Murle tribes in the camp	8th July 2013

(continued)

(continued)

Pseudonym	M/F	Ethnic group	Age	Duration of stay in the camp	Brief details	Date of interview
Chriz	M	Nuba	23	7 years	Fled insecurity in South Kordofan. Left family members there. Came to the camp to pursue an education. Completed high school in 2011 and is teaching at Kakuma secondary school	10th July 2013
Sara	F	Nuer	30	1 year	Was married as a fourth wife back in South Sudan. Living with one of the co-wives in the camp. Had run to the Reception Centre seeking shelter as a result of mistreatment from co-wife. Has one child and is pregnant. Is epileptic	4th July 2013
Atem	M	Dinka	42	21 years	Community leader. Married, with four children. Had gone back to South Sudan in 1999 to participate in the war and came back to the camp in 2005. Incentive worker with IRC. Was among 'The Lost Boys'	2nd July 2013
Paulo	M	Dinka	19	10 years	Went back to South Sudan in 2007 and came back to the camp in 2010. No parents. Living with and taking care of little brother and sister and an old relative	3rd July 2013
Jean Paul	M	Nuer	23	10 years	Fled South Sudan when unknown people attacked his village to raid cattle and every one dispersed. He was shot in the leg. Eventually learnt his parents were killed when he was reunited with his brother in 2012. Also taking care of five other children who came along with his younger brother. Does not know the whereabouts of seven of his siblings. Working in the Reconciliation committee for the Murle and the Nuer tribes in the camp	15th July 2013

(continued)

(continued)

Pseudonym	M/F	Ethnic group	Age	Duration of stay in the camp	Brief details	Date of interview
Matida	F	Nuba	28	1 month	Escaped the bombing in South Kordofan. Lost three family members. Came to the camp with three of her children, three of her sister's children, and one of her brother's children. Does not know where her husband is	4th July 2013
Juliet	F	Dinka	23	21 years	Came to the camp with mother after they were attacked by a neighbouring tribe and the father was shot dead back in South Sudan. Went back to South Sudan in 2007 but came back to the camp after receiving no help there. Husband died in an accident. Lives with her two children, mother and sister	3rd July 2013
Amuka	F	Dinka	35	14 years	Walked to Kakuma, escaping both the war in South Sudan and an abusive husband. Married again in the camp and husband died. Lives with her two children in the camp	3rd July
Okot	M	Dinka	33	21 years	Was teaching in a Special Needs nursery school in the camp but was retrenched in 2011 Doing a Laboratory course in the Camp hospital. Was among 'The Lost Boys'	2nd July 2013
Samir	M	Nuba	27	13 years	Escaped war in South Kordofan in 2000. Father fighting in the war. Went back home in 2009 but came back to the camp to continue with education. Has received counselling help and training from JRS. Community leader	8th July 2013
Pubudu	M	Nuer	20	4 years	Came to the camp when uniformed people attacked their village and family dispersed. Does not know where family members are	5th July 2013

(continued)

(continued)

Pseudonym	M/F	Ethnic group	Age	Duration of stay in the camp	Brief details	Date of interview
Rita	F	Nuba	29	1 month	Came to the camp as a result of war in South Kordofan. Father was killed and family dispersed. She does not know where her husband is. Living with her three year-old son, and is pregnant	4th July
Jerem	M	Nuba	50	7 years	Pastor of Nuban Community Church. Father died when he was seven days old. Disowned by family at 17 due to converting from Islam to Christianity. Fled from the Arabs in Sudan. Makes traditional beds for sale in the camp to raise some money	13th July 2013

References

Abu-Nimer, M. (2003). 'Toward the Theory and Practice of Positive Approaches to Peacebuilding'. In Sampson, C., Abu-Nimer, M., Liebler, C. & Whitney, D. (Eds.) *Positive Approaches to Peacebuilding: A Resource for Innovators.* Washington, D.C.: Pact Publications, pp. 13–24.

Akerlund, A. (2005). *Transforming Conflicts and Building Peace: Experience and Ideas of Swedish Civil Society Organisations.* Stockholm: SIDA.

Amollo, M.O. (2008). 'The Power of Theatre in Transforming Conflicts at Kakuma Refugee Camp'. Retrieved 11 June 2015 from: http://www.beyondintractability.org/casestudy/amollo-power.

Arendt, H. (1994). *The Origins of Totalitarianism* New York: Harcourt Books. (First published, 1951).

Audergon, A. (2008). 'Daring to Dream: Learning about Community Trauma, Accountability and Building the Future in Post-War Forums in Croatia'. In Hart, B. (Ed.) *Peacebuilding in Traumatized Societies.* Lanham: University Press of America, pp. 261–276.

Ayindo, B. (2008). 'Arts Approaches to Peace: Playing Our Way to Transcendence?' In Hart, B. (Ed.) *Peacebuilding in Traumatized Societies.* Lanham: University Press of America, pp. 185–204.

Boulding, E. (2003). 'Peace Culture for Today and Tomorrow'. In Sampson, C., Abu-Nimer, M., Liebler, C. & Whitney, D. (Eds.) *Positive Approaches to Peacebuilding: A Resource for Innovators.* Washington, D.C.: Pact Publications, pp. 83–94.

Buber, M. (1922) *The Martin Buber Reader: Essential Writings.* In Biemann, A.D. (Ed.) (2002). New York: Palgrave Macmillan.

Chupp, M. (2003). 'Creating a Culture of Peace in Postwar El Salvador'. In Sampson, C., Abu-Nimer, M., Liebler, C. & Whitney, D. (Eds.) *Positive Approaches to Peacebuilding: A Resource for Innovators.* Washington, D.C.: Pact Publications, pp. 95–118.

Gade, C.B.N. (2013) 'Ubuntu and Restorative Justice: Addressing the Strife and Divisions of the Past in Post-Apartheid South Africa'. A PhD Thesis. Aarhus University, Denmark.

Galtung, J. (1975). *Essays in Peace Research*, Volume I. Copenhagen. Christian Ejlers.

Galtung, J. (1976). 'Three Approaches to Peace: Peacekeeping, Peacemaking, and Peacebuilding'. In *Peace, War and Defense: Essays in Peace Research*, Vol. 2. pp. 297–298.

Galtung, J. (1996). *Peace by Peaceful Means: Peace and Conflict, Development and Civilization.* London: Sage.

Gebrewold, B. (2014). *'T'úmmu: An East African Perspective'.* In Dietrich, W., Alvarez, J.E., Esteva, G., Ingruber, D. & Koppensteiner, N. (Eds.) *The Palgrave International Handbook of Peace Studies: A Cultural Perspective.* New York: Palgrave, pp. 428–441.

Gobodo-Madikizela, P. (2008). 'Trauma, Forgiveness and The Witnessing Dance: Making Public Spaces Intimate'. In *Journal of Analytical Psychology* Vol. 53, pp. 169–188.

Hastrup, K. (2003). 'Violence, Suffering and Human Rights: Anthropological Reflections'. In *Anthropological Theory* Vol. 3, No. 3, pp. 309–323.

Hayes, A. & Mason, R. (2013). 'Security in Twenty-first Century Societies'. In Steiner, N; Mason, R. & Hayes, A. (Eds.) *Migration and Insecurity: Citizenship and Social Inclusion in a Transnational Era.* London: Routledge, pp. 3–16.

Herman, J. (1997). *Trauma and Recovery.* New York: Basic Books.

Humphrey, M. (2002). *The Politics of Atrocity and Reconciliation: From Terror to Trauma*, London: Routledge.

Jeong, H.-W. (1999). *Peace and Conflict Studies: An Introduction.* Aldershort, England: Ashgate Publishing.

Jeong, H.-W. (2005). *Peacebuilding in Postconflict Societies: Strategy and Process.* London: Lynne Rienner Publishers.

Kantowitz, R. & Riak, A. (2008). 'Critical Links between Peacebuilding and Trauma Healing: A Holistic Framework for Fostering Community Development'. In Hart, B. (Ed.) *Peacebuilding in Traumatized Societies.* Lanham: University Press of America, pp. 3–26.

Lederach, J.P. (1997). *Building Sustainable Peace: Sustainable Reconciliation in Divided Societies.* Washington D.C.: United States Institute of Peace Press.

Lederach, J.P. (2003). 'The Wow Factor and a Non-Theory of Change'. In Sampson, C., Abu-Nimer, M., Liebler, C. & Whitney, D. (Eds.) *Positive Approaches to Peacebuilding: A Resource for Innovators.* Washington, D.C.: Pact Publications, pp. 119–134.

Lederach, J.P. (2005). *The Moral Imagination: The Art and Soul of Building Peace.* New York: Oxford University Press.

Lederach, J.P. & Appleby, R.S. (2010). 'Strategic Peacebuilding: An Overview'. In Philpott, D. & Powers, G.F. (Eds.) *Strategies of Peace: Transforming Conflict in a Violent World.* New York: Oxford University Press, pp. 19–44.

Liebler, C. & Sampson, C. (2003). 'Appreciative Inquiry in Peacebuilding: Imagining the Possible'. In Sampson, C., Abu-Nimer, M., Liebler, C. & Whitney, D. (Eds.) *Positive Approaches to Peacebuilding: A Resource for Innovators.* Washington, D.C.: Pact Publications, pp. 55–79.

Omeje, K. (2013). 'Understanding the Diversity and Complexity of Conflict in the African Great Lakes Region'. In Omeje, K. & Hepner, T.R. (Eds.) *Conflict and Peacebuilding in the African Great Lakes Region.* Bloomington: Indiana University Press.

Opoku, K.A. (2014) '*Asomdwoe*: A West African Perspective'. In Dietrich, W., Alvarez, J.E., Esteva, G., Ingruber, D. & Koppensteiner, N. (Eds.) *The Palgrave International Handbook of Peace Studies: A Cultural Perspective.* New York: Palgrave, pp. 417–427.

Philpott, D. (2010). 'Introduction: Searching for Strategy in an Age of Peacebuilding'. In Philpott, D. & Powers, G.F. (Eds.) *Strategies of Peace: Transforming Conflict in a Violent World.* New York: Oxford University Press, pp. 3–18.

Rees, S. (2003). *Passion for Peace: Exercising Power Creatively.* Sydney: UNSW Press.

Reychler, L. (2001) 'From Conflict to Sustainable Peacebuilding: Concepts and Analytical Tools'. In Reychler, L. & Paffenholz, T. (Eds.) *Peacebuilding: A Field Guide.* Boulder: Lynne Rienner Publishers, pp. 3–15.

Rogers, C.R. (1961). *On Becoming a Person*. Boston: Houghton Mifflin.
Scarry, E. (1985). *The Body in Pain: The Making and Unmaking of the World.* Oxford: Oxford University Press.
Schirch, L. (2004). *The Little Book of Strategic Peacebuilding*. Intercourse, PA: Good Books.
Schirch, L. (2005). *Ritual and Symbol in Peacebuilding.* Bloomfield, CT: Kumarian Press.
Senehi, J. & Byrne, S. (2011). 'Where do We Go From Here?' In Philpott, D. & Powers, G.F. (Eds.) *Strategies of Peace: Transforming Conflict in a Violent World.* New York: Oxford University Press, pp. 397–403.
Sider, N.G. (2003). 'Transcendence: Discovering Resources for Posttraumatic Healing and Growth'. In Sampson, C., Abu-Nimer, M., Liebler, C. & Whitney, D. (Eds.) *Positive Approaches to Peacebuilding: A Resource for Innovators.* Washington, D.C.: Pact Publications, pp. 287–314.
Staub, E., Pearlman, L.A., Bilali, R. (2008). 'Psychological Recovery, Reconciliation and the Prevention of New Violence: An Approach and Its Uses in Rwanda'. In Hart, B. (Ed.) *Peacebuilding in Traumatized Societies.* Lanham: University Press of America, pp. 131–154.
UNHCR (2005). 'UNHCR's official voluntary repatriation of refugees to South Sudan to start Saturday'. Retrieved 11 June 2015 from: http://www.unhcr.org/43a679bd4.html.
Van der Merwe, H. & Vienings, T. (2001). 'Coping With Trauma'. In Reychler, L. & Paffenholz, T. (Eds.) *Peacebuilding: A Field Guide*. Boulder: Lynne Rienner Publishers, pp. 343–351.
Vasilevska, B. (2014). 'The Role of Settlement Agencies in Promoting Refugee Resilience'. In Simich, L. & Andermann, L. (Eds.) *Refuge and Resilience: International Perspectives on Migration*. New York: Springer, pp. 167–181.
Whitney, D., Liebler, C. & Cooperrider, D. (2003). 'Appreciative Inquiry in Organizations and International Development: An Invitation to Share and Learn Across Fields'. In Sampson, C., Abu-Nimer, M., Liebler, C. & Whitney, D. (Eds.) *Positive Approaches to Peacebuilding: A Resource for Innovators.* Washington, D.C.: Pact Publications, pp. 25–54.
Williams, S. (2001). 'The Usefulness of Humor'. In Reychler, L. & Paffenholz, T. (Eds.) *Peacebuilding: A Field Guide*. Boulder: Lynne Rienner Publishers. pp. 492–496.

Chapter 7
Conclusion: The Journey Continues

Yet, today I call you to my riverside,
If you will study war no more. Come,
Clad in peace and I will sing the songs
The Creator gave to me when I and the
Tree and the stone were one...
The River sang and sings on.
Maya Angelou, 'On the Pulse of the Morning', 1993

7.1 The Other Side of the River

In Talia's next dream, she found she had finally crossed the river, and was standing at the edge on the other side! The journey across the river had not been easy. Her pursuer, and many others, old and young, from different sides of the warring tribes, had joined them in the safety boat. The journey took many days, and the waters were turbulent most of the time. On a few occasions, a crocodile reared its head near their boat threatening to attack, but they had concertedly struck the animal with sticks, poles, and oars, and sometimes used the very weapons they had used against one another on the other side of the river. They were all called upon to row the boat to safety, a number of them in turn, and they had to learn how to do it right and arrange appropriate schedules that worked for everyone. The owners of the boat could not provide enough food for everyone, and Talia and her companions had to share the little they had and take particular care for the oldest, the weakest and youngest. The owners of the boat were focused on getting the boat to the other side. They had to be right on schedule. Talia and her companions sang songs, told stories of their past experiences, and created new stories of what they imagined could be. Finally they got to the other side. Talia found herself standing on the edge of the river, looking ahead, at the expansive plain that spread out before her. This was not the end after all! She and her companions were only just beginning another journey...

L.W. Gitau, *Trauma-Sensitivity and Peacebuilding*, The Anthropocene: Politik—Economics—Society—Science 12, DOI 10.1007/978-3-319-49803-4_7

7.2 The Encounter

In tracing the journey of the South Sudanese survivors of conflict and mass violence from their country of origin to Kakuma refugee camp, we encounter the various ways in which the survivors experienced the consequences of the war, back in South Sudan, on their journey to the camp, and now in the camp. Of particular note is the pain of witnessing loved ones being tortured and killed, and the associated dehumanization in the hands of the perpetrators, the separation from loved ones and resultant loneliness, and the loss of security that forced the survivors to flee for refuge in Kakuma. The long journey the survivors took seeking refuge, which was not uniform but rather tended to take divergent forms for different refugees, was also seen as a journey in search of the identity they lost in leaving their country of origin and being deprived of citizenship. This was seen in their desire to identify with the notion of 'The Lost Boys' who gained much acclaim from their story of having walked for very long distances in search of refuge, and a recognized and respected identity.

Within the camp, the refugees were found to continue to experience distressing circumstances, as disease and death continued to be a reality, as well as scarcity of provisions. In this respect, some of the survivors seemed to have lost all vitality of life and seemed to be drifting along, resigned to whatever may come their way. Dependency on UNHCR for all provisions, despondency attitudes, and a lack of agency ensued in these survivors. These, combined with the PTSD symptoms portrayed by some of the survivors in the form of intrusive memories of their past pain, torture and killing of loved ones, as well as avoidance of the happenings, made it very difficult to envision the possibility of peacebuilding and the realization of peace for the survivors. As Talia and her companions experienced in the dream *… the waters were turbulent most of the time … a crocodile reared its head near their boat threatening to attack …*

Further, we encounter the gendered ways in which the participants of this study were impacted by the traumatic experiences, and how these gendered ways complicated the path to peacebuilding for the survivors. The threat and experience of rape for the women survivors in particular marked a significant meandering of their path to peace. UNHCR and its partnering agencies are not adequately able to protect the women survivors in the camp from the threat of rape. Further, the identity of these women survivors is subsumed in their label as refugee women, thus rendering them vulnerable and unable to express their other identities as they negotiate their path to peace. The interconnectedness of rape with conflict and mass violence further tends to treat rape in war and rape in peace as two separate entities, seemingly suggesting that rape in certain circumstances is not as atrocious a crime, as in others. Yet, rape at all times is a human rights violation aimed at degrading the victim's identity, dominating and dehumanising her. The threat and occurrence of rape in war mixes up with other traumas experienced by survivors of conflict and mass violence thus further complicating the terrain of the journey to peace.

The disruption of the family systems as a result of death and separation of members of family units led to disorganization and reorganization of the traditional roles of different members of the family. Death in war had for instance resulted in high numbers of widows in the camp, who had to take up roles traditionally held by men, such as constructing houses for their families. Further, the dependency on UNHCR for food rations in the camp had disrupted the dynamic of men fending for their families, resulting in a feeling of uselessness that led some men to seek solace in illicit brew in the camp. As a consequence, more and more women had taken on the responsibility of taking care of their families in the camp, demonstrating a role reversal. The gendered effects are thus interwoven with the effects of the traumatic experiences on the culture of the South Sudanese, forming an overarching situation in which the survivors find themselves disoriented and unable to meet the challenges of peacebuilding.

On examining the interventions the South Sudanese survivors of the conflict received in Kakuma to cope with their traumatic experiences, we find that interventions that are trauma- and culture-sensitive, taking into consideration the complex and multifaceted ways in which the survivors experienced and responded to the traumatic events, contribute to helping the survivors in recovery from trauma, prevent a recurrence of violence, and help facilitate peacebuilding. Trauma-sensitivity in the process of offering basic necessities such as food, shelter and health facilities in the camp entails a recognition that the basic necessities are important in recovery for the survivors not only at the physical level, but the psychological level as well. The manner in which the basic necessities are offered to the survivors is therefore of crucial importance and may serve to either accentuate the survivors' feelings of helplessness and eventual apathy, or may help to empower and encourage them on the path to peace.

Trauma-sensitivity involves taking into consideration the ways in which the interventions serve to humanize, where the survivors were dehumanized, rebuild connections where they were destroyed by violence and displacement, and restore a sense of belonging, meaning and purpose where these were shattered during the mass violence. This sensitivity involves a recognition of the social realities of the survivors, including the gendered ways in which they are affected in receiving the interventions.

Further, interventions offered to the survivors in the camp may be more effective if they are cognizant of, and promote the capacity of the survivors to recover and be well on the path to peacebuilding. This capacity is found in some of the participants who portrayed a positive attitude, reliance on community support, a long term vision and mission, selflessness, faith in God, personal initiative and agency, and inner strength. These interconnected aspects denote resilience in these participants who were able to withstand the negative consequences of their traumatic experiences, bounce back and demonstrate enthusiasm, commitment and engagement in productive tasks, and thrive. Of particular relevance to the South Sudanese refugees is the concept of community resilience, which resonates with the community-oriented ways in which they experience life. Community resilience is understood to mean a community's capacity to withstand collective trauma, identify and mobilize its resources to cope with traumatic experiences and engage in positive outcomes, which include peacebuilding activities. In the dream, Talia and her companions had *concertedly struck the animal with sticks, poles, and oars, and sometimes used the very weapons they had used against one another on the other side of the river.*

On reflecting on the participants' perceptions and definitions of peace, we find that some participants conceive of peace as an assumed state, meaning that it is nonexistent in reality, and its seeming appearance is devoid of substance. This peace has the characteristics of avoiding the real state of things and dwelling on the surface. It sometimes takes the form of the officially constructed peace, and manifests as peaceful co-existence amongst warring groups. The emptiness of this peace demonstrates the gap that needs to be filled in envisioning peace for the survivors of conflict and mass violence. This emptiness is reminiscent of the empty void experienced and expressed by some of the participants in relating their traumatic experiences. The emptiness however does not discourage the participants of this study from being part of this peace. An exploration of the assumed peace as described by the participants revealed that there is value in this type of peace, empty as it may seem, insofar as it translates into an imagination of what peace can look like, if it were real. An imagined peace can translate into a possible, real peace, if efforts are made to make the imagined concrete.

Advancing on the path to peace reveals the ineptness of isolation and the efficacy of relationships with others, for steady progress on the journey. Relationships are seen to be the core of peacebuilding. The stories most of the participants told about their experiences of trauma, the interventions they had received, and their perceptions of peace, emphasized the interconnectedness of the survivors with one another. Martin Buber's 'I-Thou' concept, and the African perspectives of peace discussed, all underscore the centrality of relationships in understanding peace and implementing peacebuilding. Considering the culturally-embedded ways in which people experience reality, this centrality of relationships reveals the community-oriented ways in which the South Sudanese experienced their lives, and consequently points to the appropriateness of community-oriented interventions to help the survivors work through their traumatic experiences.

A further exploration reveals the connection between relationships and the recovery from trauma. Recovery from trauma takes place in the context of relationships, as the survivor is helped to re-create the capacities of trust, initiative, competence and identity that were shattered during the traumatic event, through renewed connections with other people. This restoration of the survivors' previously shattered capacities is found to contribute to their ability to engage in peacebuilding activities, which correspondingly depend on relationships in terms of community mobilization and participation, for their success.

It emerges that this journey towards understanding of the role of trauma-sensitivity in peacebuilding is a journey towards discovery of what comprises 'a whole life, complete life' for the survivors, as Patrick,[1] one of the participants in the research, remarked in defining peace. The various aspects of this 'complete life' for the survivors, which include security, citizenship, and freedom from direct, structural and cultural violence, are all intertwined with the traumas the survivors of conflict and mass violence experience. Thus, in considering interventions that are trauma-sensitive, addressing these aspects becomes essential. This calls for the application of a wide array of approaches to effectively address the various aspects, and points to the continuous nature of the path of discovery of what would work for the best interests of the survivors of conflict and mass violence. The exploratory journey continues.

The efforts and possibilities of making the imagined peace concrete are identified further in the participants' expressions of hope and courage, which entail going beyond the conventional, the experienced and the known. On exploration of some of the participants' perceptions, taking steps to go beyond the conventional image of the vulnerable, dependent and helpless refugee revealed the resilient individual who believed that she could make it against all odds, overcome and prevail over her traumatic experiences, and emerge as an enthusiastic, committed and productive member of her community, ready to help others. This discovery presents a possibility of going beyond an imagined peace to a possible, real, peace.

This exploratory journey also involves taking a risk and stepping out into the unknown, and leaving room for the unexpected to happen along the way. Some participants demonstrated this courage, through their faith and determination, and hope that things would turn out positive. There is value in taking this risk and daring to imagine making a difference by embracing the traumas experienced and working with what has been suffered to craft a better, more peaceful future. Interventions that demonstrate and encourage taking this valuable risk are seen to be trauma-sensitive.

An appreciation of the complex and differentiated realities of the survivors, and adapting a holistic integrated approach in the interventions they receive is seen to have potential to facilitate sustainable peace. Aligning the interventions to the realities of the survivors is considered to be a demonstration of respect for the survivors as individuals, and to protect their human dignity.

Further, an adventurous turn in the exploration of these possibilities considers the potential for transformation that is achievable through the creative arts. The arts are seen to take the survivors, and all of us who are concerned, beyond what is experienced to what is desired, in this case peace. By employing symbolic acts and rituals, and drawing on the culture of the South Sudanese which is rich in dance, drama, music and poetry, interventions can go beyond what the survivors have experienced and expressed, reinstate meaning where it has been lost, dramatize possibilities where none seem apparent, and contribute to a transformation from an assumption to a reality of peace. *Talia and her companions sang songs, told stories of their past experiences, and created new stories of what they imagined could be.*

[1]Interview with Patrick, KRM43 on 15 and 16 July 2013. See Appendix 7.1.

7.3 The Discovery

There is need to revisit the theoretical basis of the provision of these interventions. It is particularly important to put into detailed consideration *what* traumatic experiences the survivors have gone through, and *how* they have experienced them, in designing and providing interventions for the survivors. The scope of understanding these experiences, and the manner in which they are experienced, determine the extent to which the interventions provided for the survivors facilitate peacebuilding. A lack of sensitivity to the trauma experienced by the survivors and how they experience it leads to interventions that are at best removed, and at worst detrimental to the welfare of the survivors. The various interventions should thus not be seen as compartmentalized, each working on its own to meet a particular need, but all functioning together to help the survivor towards experiencing peace.

This argument is consistent with Hart's (2008) conception of the 'Peacebuilding Wheel' discussed in Chap. 2. The wheel consists of 'tangible' elements such as food, shelter, infrastructure and peace agreements, and 'intangible' elements such as psychological and spiritual needs, and Hart argues that the tangible elements need to be seen to have psychological importance if they are to contribute to peacebuilding. Trauma-sensitivity is necessary in attending to the tangible elements of the peacebuilding wheel, for peace to be sustainable.

The argument is also consistent with Yoder's (2013) concept of being trauma-informed in working with trauma survivors, which entails being cognizant of the multifaceted and culturally-embedded ways survivors are impacted by trauma, and the need to engage different approaches in addressing this trauma. We see how survivors are impacted by the traumatic experiences in differentiated ways, and the relationship of the interventions they receive to their recovery from trauma and engagement in peacebuilding. This book adds to the repertoire of other studies exploring the landscape of the link between mental health and psychosocial support services and peacebuilding.

The discorvery disrupts the conventional image of the refugee. As argued by various authors in refugee studies and discussed in this book, the image of the refugee presented to the world is one of 'the suffering stranger' (Butt 2002: 6), a person 'reduced to bare life' (Agamben 1998: 171), the individual 'deprived of citizenship and dependent on the goodwill and moral responsibility of strangers' (Humphrey 2002: 118), 'helpless and vulnerable' (Harrell-Bond 1999: 153), and as a group, 'homogeneous, undifferentiated masses' (Harrell-Bond 1999: 140). Listening to the stories of the survivors, about their lives before coming to the camp, the traumatic experiences that led them to come to the camp, and their lives in the camp, reveals individuals who are beyond the label of 'refugee' placed on them, and whose lives take on diverse and deep meanings in other contexts besides the refugee context.

Sadly, their identities have been subsumed by this refugee label, which makes it difficult for them to express their other identities and complicates negotiating the challenges that they face. Their status as refugees requires of them to be suffering, deprived, helpless and vulnerable. Yet, the exploration of the ways the participants of the research coped with traumatic experiences reveals the resilience portrayed by some of them in their attitude, faith, community engagement, having a vision and taking personal initiative. The ability to step beyond the conventional and the expected, and a willingness to take the risk to step into the unknown, reveals the potential for peacebuilding that the survivors have.

The discovery further reveals a symbiotic relationship between traumatic experiences of survivors of conflict and mass violence, recovery from trauma, peacebuilding and peace. It establishes relationships as the nexus, as shown in Fig. 7.1.

From the stories they told during the interviews, it emerges that the survivors were living in a state of relative peace before violence erupted in their country of origin. One of the key traumatic experiences the participants of the research related, as discussed in Chap. 4, was the separation from loved ones, sometimes through death, and sometimes after members of families dispersed to different locations for safety. The disconnection with loved ones resulted in a sense of disorientation, thus underscoring the importance of relationships in their lives. To recover from this sense of disconnection and disorientation and begin to make meaning of their lives once again, correspondingly depends on making renewed connections. This is seen in the participants' emphasis on community support in discussing the interventions to cope with traumatic experiences, and the relevance of a community-oriented model of intervention as discussed in Chap. 5. The recovery from trauma, predominantly based on the reestablished connections, helps restore the survivors' capacities for productive activities, which include engagement in peacebuilding. Peacebuilding is similarly seen to rely heavily on the synergetic energy of relationships. Finally peace itself is perceived as relationship, as seen in the participants' expressions in defining peace, discussed in Chap. 6. This centrality of relationships is key to the link between trauma and peacebuilding.

Fig. 7.1 The Nexus: Relationships. *Source* The author

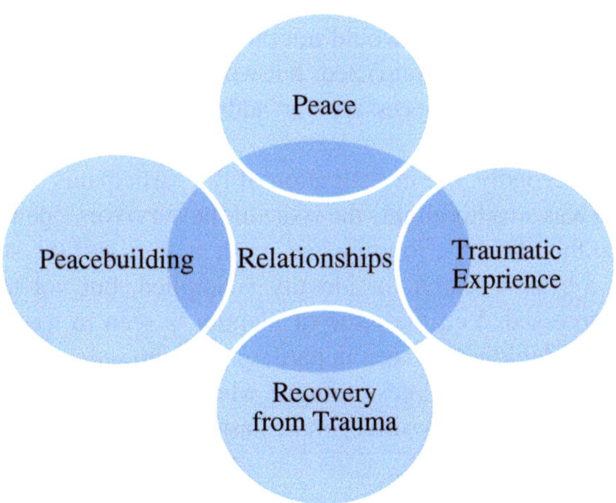

Policies applied by groups and organizations working with survivors of conflict and mass violence could benefit from a specific attention to the survivors, their particular experiences of trauma, and their perceptions of what works best for them, in envisioning a future of peace. This involves seeking to grasp the experiential world of the participants and how they are making sense of it. The search reveals the complex and diverse ways the survivors are impacted by the traumatic events, and how the type of interventions and manner of provision of these interventions need to be sensitive to these realities.

Further, a focus on the survivors, letting them tell their story, allows for surprises and lets the survivors who go beyond the orthodox image of the vulnerable, helpless and dependent refugee to emerge. It also allows opportunity for the potential for peacebuilding that exists in these resilient survivors to be realized. Thus, groups and organizations working for peacebuilding in the context of mass violence could benefit from programs that emphasize trauma-awareness, encourage capacities for resilience in the survivors, engage the arts in peacebuilding to help go beyond what the survivors have experienced, underscore the centrality of relationships, and employ a variety of approaches to address the wide range of aspects that entail peace for the survivors.

7.4 Future Journeys

In exploring the gendered ways in which the participants are impacted by the traumatic experiences, it emerges that there is a limited focus on the ways in which men in particular were impacted. Many authors exploring the landscape of conflict and mass violence focus extensively on women, particularly on the topic of rape in war. While this focus is understandable, especially given the egregious nature of rape as a human rights violation both in war and in peace, an investigation of the ways men are particularly impacted and the ramifications of the findings to the work of peacebuilding after mass violence is worthwhile, as a topic for future research. This investigation would not only serve to balance the apparent particular focus on how women are impacted, but would also be an important contribution to the array of approaches necessary for addressing the various aspects of peace after mass violence.

Secondly, the investigation of the participants' literal journey from South Sudan to Kakuma highlights the issue of the survivors' identity with an interesting allusion to the effect the journey had on their feet, and the story of The Lost Boys. In this way, their search for identity is implied, but not thoroughly explored or clearly expressed. Yet, the issue of identity is seen to have ramifications for the work of peacebuilding, as seen in participants who seemed to have taken up the identity of a resigned and helpless refugee who needs to be rescued, in contrast to those who exuded a more positive, enthusiastic view of themselves. It would be worthwhile to investigate in more detail, in further research, this search for and formation of the survivors' identity.

Related to the topic of identity is the overarching concern of the gap that exists between the survivors of mass violence (the helped), and the interveners (the helpers). This book has shown that this yawning gap continues to threaten the possibilities of envisioning and realizing a peace for the survivors, insofar as the 'Us' versus 'Them' mentality prevails. This gap allows for the perception of the realities of the survivors as removed from, and unidentifiable with, the realities of those offering the interventions. As such, it seems the two groups are operating on two different sides of humanity, rather than on one which they share in actual sense. This gap is particularly visible when one considers the existence and expansion of the humanitarian industry, which seems to thrive on the presence and upsurge of victims of violence. Beyond revealing the existence of this gap and some of the ramifications it has for peacebuilding, this book did not address how this gap can be alleviated. Further research can investigate the nature of this gap, and explore ways of closing it, to allow for deeper possibilities of peacebuilding.

Peacebuilding mechanisms aimed at the macro-level and focusing on the economic, political and security structures while paying little or no attention to the micro-level psychosocial approaches have proven to be inadequate in situations of conflict and mass violence and peace has remained elusive for survivors of mass violence, as the case of South Sudanese refugees in Kakuma demonstrates. This inadequacy has highlighted the need to shift focus and explore mechanisms that pay more attention to the people most directly affected by the violence. This shift is particularly notable in the growing field of Mental Health and Psychosocial Support (MHPSS) and its link to peacebuilding.

With this regard, this book has explored the interventions that the South Sudanese refugees in Kakuma receive, and the link of these interventions to peacebuilding. The book has identified trauma-sensitivity as a significant element in the interventions, and demonstrated how trauma-sensitivity in the interventions the survivors receive, supports peacebuilding. This sensitivity entails taking into consideration the complex and multifaceted ways in which the survivors experience and respond to the traumatic events, encouraging capacities for resilience in the survivors, engaging the creative arts, and emphasising the centrality of relationships.

In this way, this book contributes to the identification of the various pieces of the puzzle that are needed for building sustainable peace after mass violence. There are more pieces to the puzzle. A new journey of exploration is called for. As Talia observed when she got to the other side of the river, looked ahead and saw the expansive plain spreading out before her, *this was not the end after all! She and her companions were only just beginning another journey...*

Appendix 7.1

Pseudonym	M/F	Ethnic group	Age	Duration of stay in the camp	Brief details	Date of interview
Patrick	M	Murle	40	5 months	People from the Nuer Community attacked his village and killed many people, his wife and children ran to the bush where his wife delivered their last child. SPLA soldiers attacked his village, many people were killed and he sustained injuries. Worked as a Livestock officer. In the Reconciliation committee between the Murle and the Nuer in the camp	15th and 16th July 2013

References

Agamben, G. (1998). *Homo Sacer: Sovereign Power and Bare Life*. Stanford: Stanford University Press.

Butt, L. (2002). 'The Suffering Stranger: Medical Anthropology and International Morality'. In *Medical Anthropology* Vol. 21 No. 1, pp. 1–24.

Harrell-Bond, B. (1999). 'The Experience of Refugees as Recipients of Aid'. In Ager, A. (Ed.) *Refugees: Perspectives on the Experience of Forced Migration*. London: Continuum, pp. 136–168.

Hart, B. (2008). 'Introduction'. In Hart, B. (Ed.) *Peacebuilding in Traumatized Societies*. New York: University Press of America, pp. vii–xi.

Humphrey, M. (2002). 'Humanitarianism, Terrorism and the Transnational Border'. *Social Analysis*. Vol. 46. No. 1, pp. 117–122.

Yoder, C. (2013). 'Trauma-Sensitive Development and Humanitarian Aid'. In *Peacebuilder*. Eastern Mennonite University: Centre for Justice and Peacebuilding, pp. 1–2. Retrieved 13 July 2015 from: http://emu.edu/now/peacebuilder/2013/03/trauma-sensitive-acknowledging-peoples-difficult-experiences-can-help-them-move-forward/.

The International Peace Research Association (IPRA)

Founded in 1964, the *International Peace Research Association* (IPRA) developed from a conference organised by the Quaker International Conferences and Seminars in Clarens, Switzerland, 16–20 August 1963. The participants decided to hold international Conferences on Research on International Peace and Security (COROIPAS), which would be organised by a Continuing Committee similar to the Pugwash Conferences. Under the leadership of John Burton, the Continuing Committee met in London, 1–3 December 1964. At that time, they took steps to broaden the original concept of holding research conferences. The decision was made to form a professional association with the principal aim of increasing the quantity of research focused on world peace and ensuring its scientific quality.

An Executive Committee including Bert V.A. Roling, Secretary General (The Netherlands), John Burton (United Kingdom), Ljubivoje Acimovic (Yugoslavia), Jerzy Sawicki (Poland), and Johan Galtung (Norway) was appointed. This group was also designated as Nominating Committee for a 15-person Advisory Council to be elected at the first general conference of IPRA, to represent various regions, disciplines, and research interests in developing the work of the Association. Since then, IPRA has held 26 biennial general conferences, the venues of which were chosen with a view to reflecting the association's global scope.

IPRA, the global network of peace researchers, held its 25th General Conference on the occasion of its 50th anniversary in Istanbul, Turkey in August 2014, when peace researchers from all parts of the world had the opportunity to exchange actionable knowledge on the conference theme of 'Uniting for sustainable peace and universal values'. The 26th IPRA General Conference took place between 28 November and 1 December 2016 in Freetown, Sierra Leone on the theme: Agenda for Peace and Development: Conflict Prevention, Post-Conflict Transformation, and the Conflict, Disaster and Development Debate.
On IPRA http://www.iprapeace.org/.

On Previous IPRA General Conferences

IPRA 2012 in Mie, Japan https://www.facebook.com/media/set/?set=a.321841277928978.77587.320866028026503&type=3.
IPRA 2014 in Istanbul, Turkey https://www.facebook.com/ipra2014.

L.W. Gitau, *Trauma-Sensitivity and Peacebuilding*, The Anthropocene: Politik—Economics—Society—Science 12, DOI 10.1007/978-3-319-49803-4

IPRA 2016 in Freetown, Sierra Leone http://www.iprapeace.org/images/newsletters/IPRA2016FreetownCONFERENCEBROCHURE.pdf.

IPRA's Scientific Commissions

Between the biannual conferences the major scientific work is done by IPRA's Commissions. For details see: http://www.iprapeace.org/index.php/commissions-commitees/ipra-commissions.

IPRA's Regional Organisations

IPRA has five Regional Organisations

- **Asia-Pacific Peace Research Association (APPRA)** http://appra.net/about/.
- **Africa Peace Research and Education Association (AFPREA)**
- **European Peace Research Association (EUPRA)** http://euprapeace.org/eupra/.
- **Latin American Peace Research Association (CLAIP)** http://www.crim.unam.mx/claip/inicio.
- **Peace and Justice Studies Association (North America)** http://www.peacejusticestudies.org/.

IPRA's Conferences, Secretary Generals and Presidents 1964–2018

IPRA General Conferences	IPRA Secretary Generals/Presidents
1. Groningen, The Netherlands (1965)	1964–1971 Bert V. A. Roling (the Netherlands)
2. Tallberg, Sweden (1967)	1971–1975 Asbjorn Eide (Norway)
3. Karlovy Vary, Czechoslovakia (1969)	1975–1979 Raimo Väyrynen (Finland)
4. Bled, Yugoslavia (1971)	1979–1983 Yoshikazu Sakamoto (Japan)
5. Varanasi, India (1974)	1983–1987 Chadwick Alger (USA)
6. Turku, Finland (1975)	1987–1989 Clovis Brigagão (Brazil)
7. Oaxtepec, Mexico (1977)	1989–1991 Elise Bouding (USA)
8. Königstein, FRG (1979)	1991–1994 Paul Smoker (USA)
9. Orillia, Canada (1981)	1995–1997 Karlheinz Koppe (Germany)
10. Győr, Hungary (1983)	1997–2000 Bjørn Møller (Denmark)
11. Sussex, England (1986)	2000–2005 Katsuya Kodama (Japan)
12. Rio de Janeiro, Brazil (1988)	2005–2009 Luc Reychler (Belgium)
13. Groningen, The Netherlands (1990)	2009–2012 Jake Lynch (UK/Australia) and Katsuya Kodama (Japan)
14. Kyoto, Japan (1992)	2012–2016 Nesrin Kenar (Turkey) and Ibrahim Shaw (Sierra Leone/UK)
15. Valletta, Malta (1994)	2016–2018 Úrsula Oswald Spring (Mexico) and Katsuya Kodama (Japan)
16. Brisbane, Australia (1996)	**IPRA Presidents**
17. Durban, South Africa (1998)	The first IPRA President was Kevin Clements (New Zealand/USA, 1994–1998)
18. Tampere, Finland (2000)	His successor was Úrsula Oswald Spring (Mexico, 1998–2000)
19. Suwon, Korea (2002)	
20. Sopron, Hungary (2004)	
21. Calgary, Canada (2006)	
22. Leuven, Belgium (2008)	
23. Sydney, Australia (2010)	
24. Mie, Japan (2012)	
25. Istanbul, Turkey (2014)	
26. Freetown, Sierra Leone (2016)	
27. NN (2018)	

The Department of Peace and Conflict Studies, University of Sydney, Australia

The University of Sydney's Department of Peace and Conflict Studies promotes interdisciplinary research and teaching on the causes of conflict and the conditions that affect conflict resolution and peace. Research projects and other activities focus on the resolution of conflict with a view to attaining just societies.

The Department aims to facilitate dialogue between individuals, groups or communities who are concerned with conditions of positive peace, whether in interpersonal relationships, community relations, within organisations and nations, or with reference to international relations.

The Department is involved with the selection and awarding of the Sydney Peace Prize since 1998. Its most recent recipient in 2016 was human rights and climate change activist and author Naomi Klein. Previous recipients of this prestigious award include Archbishop Desmond Tutu (1999), Vandana Shiva (2010), Xanana Gusmao (2000) and Australian Indigenous rights leader Patrick Dobson (2008).

Other projects with which the Department of Peace and Conflict Studies includes the establishment of an Australian Peace Museum.

Profile and details of The University of Sydney Department of Peace and Conflict Studies is available from: http://sydney.edu.au/arts/peace_conflict/.

L.W. Gitau, *Trauma-Sensitivity and Peacebuilding*, The Anthropocene: Politik—Economics—Society—Science 12, DOI 10.1007/978-3-319-49803-4

About the Author

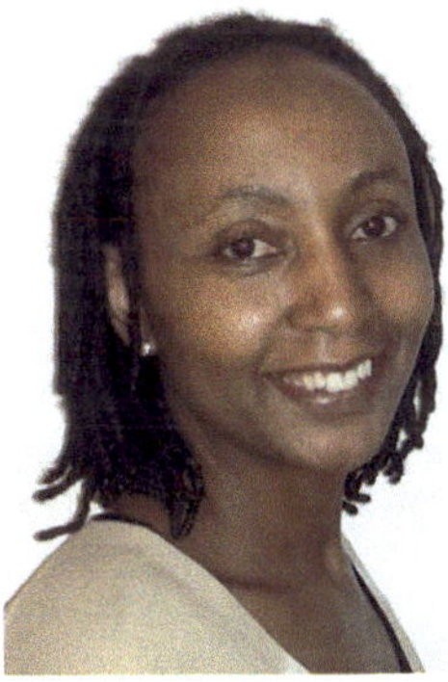

Dr. Lydia Wanja Gitau (Kenya) is a graduate of the Centre for Peace and Conflict Studies, University of Sydney. She was the recipient of the 2014–2015 IPRA Foundation's Dorothy M. Senesh Graduate Fellowship, and the 2014 Postgraduate Teaching Fellowship of the Faculty of Arts and Social Sciences, University of Sydney. Her employment history includes lecturing at Kenya Methodist University and counselling at Jomo Kenyatta University in Kenya. She has been a part-time lecturer and tutor at University of Sydney and University of Technology Sydney (UTS). She is currently working at the NSW Service for the Treatment and Rehabilitation of Torture and Trauma Survivors (STARTTS). She lives in Sydney with her husband and two children. This book is a revised version of Lydia's Ph.D. thesis. She is interested in examining the post-conflict interventions that have potential to support long-lasting peace in the African Region and beyond, with a particular focus on trauma-sensitive interventions.

Among Lydia's peer-reviewed publications are: (with Paul Rhodes, 2016) '"A Dark Stone in My Stomach": Interventions for Survivors of Mass Violence and Building Sustainable Peace', *Journal of Peacebuilding and Development* Vol. 11. No. 3, pp. 37–52; (with Wendy Lambourne, 2013): 'Psychosocial Interventions, Peacebuilding and Development in Rwanda', *Journal of Peacebuilding and Development* Vol. 8 No. 3; Book Review of War to Peace Transition: Conflict Intervention and Peacebuilding in Liberia. Edited by Kenneth Omeje. Published in *Journal of Peacebuilding and Development*, November 2009.

Among her non-refereed articles are: 'The Power of the Afflicted', *PeaceWrite*s, 2013/2 October 2014, Centre for Peace and Conflict Studies, University of Sydney, Australia. 'Where is Hope? Rakela in Kakuma', *PeaceWrites*, 2013/2 October 2013, Centre for Peace and Conflict Studies, University of Sydney, Australia; 'Kenya Learns to Walk at 50', *PeaceWrites*, 2013/1 May 2013, Centre for Peace and Conflict Studies, University of Sydney, Australia; 'Oily Peace in South Sudan',

L.W. Gitau, *Trauma-Sensitivity and Peacebuilding*, The Anthropocene: Politik—Economics—Society—Science 12, DOI 10.1007/978-3-319-49803-4

PeaceWrites, 2012/2 October 2012, Centre for Peace and Conflict Studies, University of Sydney, Australia.

Lydia has presented conference papers on: 'Peace in My Father's World: Trauma Sensitivity in Interventions for Survivors of Conflict and Mass Violence' at the 38th African Studies Association of Australasia and the Pacific (AFSAAP), Deakin University, Melbourne, 28–30 October 2015; (with Wendy Lambourne) 'Rwanda 20 Years On: Trauma, Transitional Justice and Reconciliation After Genocide' at the International Network of Genocide Scholars Fourth Global Conference on Genocide, Cape Town, 4–7 December 2014; 'Beyond Hope: Trauma and Resilience in South Sudanese Refugees in Kakuma Refugee Camp, Kenya' at the International Peace Research Association (IPRA) Conference, Sakarya University, Istanbul, Turkey, 12 August 2014; 'Blurred by Pain: Trauma Healing and Social Justice for Survivors of Mass Violence' at the Higher Degree Research Conference on Social Justice, Division of Humanities and Social Sciences, 27 November 2013, University of Sydney, Australia; 'Trauma Healing for Peace and Development: Considering South Sudan' at the 2nd Annual Interdisciplinary Conference from 25–29 June 2013, Catholic University of Eastern Africa, Nairobi, Kenya; 'Resilience in Survivors of Mass Violence and Its Contribution to Reconciliation in Post-Conflict Rwanda' at the 35th African Studies Association of Australasia and the Pacific (AFSAAP), 26–29 November, 2012, Australian National University, Canberra, Australia.

Address Dr. Lydia Wanja Gitau.
Email lydia.gitau@sydney.edu.au.
Webpage http://sydney.edu.au/arts/peace_conflict/people/lydia_gitau.shtml.

Index

L.W. Gitau, *Trauma-Sensitivity and Peacebuilding*, The Anthropocene: Politik—Economics—Society—Science 12, DOI 10.1007/978-3-319-49803-4

MIX
Papier aus verantwortungsvollen Quellen
Paper from responsible sources
FSC® C105338

If you have any concerns about our products,
you can contact us on
ProductSafety@springernature.com

In case Publisher is established outside the EU,
the EU authorized representative is:
Springer Nature Customer Service Center GmbH
Europaplatz 3, 69115 Heidelberg, Germany

Printed by Libri Plureos GmbH
in Hamburg, Germany